Praise for

Believing Me

"Ingrid's book is a lyrical and deeply authentic memoir of trauma, complex post-trauma, and narcissistic abuse. She provides that rarest of things, a realistic glimpse into the evolution of healing in a survivor, and humanizes a painful journey that has too often been simplified. Her story is compelling and she shares it with compassion, vulnerability and honesty. This book should be required reading for anyone who wants to learn about complex trauma, narcissistic family systems, and the landscape of healing from trauma. All survivors will see a part of themselves in Ingrid's story."

— Dr. Ramani Durvasula
Clinical psychologist, author, and professor emerita of psychology. Founder and CEO of LUNA Education, Training and Consulting.

"Gorgeously told, *Believing Me* is a gripping, courageous memoir of healing from a deeply compassionate clinician—and a powerful invitation to heal."

— Dr. Craig Malkin
Author of the internationally acclaimed *Rethinking Narcissism*, clinical psychologist, and lecturer for Harvard Medical School.

"Dr. Ingrid Clayton demonstrates just how powerful the writing process can be in trauma recovery. I am most grateful that she is allowing us as readers to share the journey with her. Ingrid is full of candor and insight, and her vulnerability is a true gift to the helping professions and trauma survivors alike."

— **Dr. Jamie Marich**

Founder, The Institute for Creative Mindfulness EMDR Trainer and author, including *Trauma and the 12 Steps: An Inclusive Guide to Enhancing Your Recovery.*

"A gripping, page-turning memoir about what happens when the adults who are supposed to protect us do the opposite. Ingrid Clayton was a victim of gas-lighting that began in her pre-teen years and persisted for over thirty years. Despite being a therapist and seeing multiple therapists, Clayton had to learn that her trauma was not in the past and no one could free her from it other than herself."

— **Dr. Paria Hassouri**

Pediatrician and author of *Found in Transition: A Mother's Evolution during her Child's Gender Change.*

"This beautifully written memoir illustrates Dr. Clayton's courage in healing herself from her childhood trauma. In my many years as a Dialectical Behavioral Therapy researcher and clinician, this is the first account I have read describing the application of DBT treatment principles to heal complex trauma from pervasive childhood invalidation. Childhood invalidation is an insidious trauma that is difficult to treat, requiring strategies beyond regular talk therapy. This book is a unique and invaluable resource for DBT therapists, therapists more generally, and patients who are longing to heal."

— Dr. Milton Brown
Clinical psychologist, professor, director of the DBT Center of San Diego, and author of the upcoming book, *A Long Way From Home: A Memoir on Overcoming Traumatic Grief.*

Believing Me

Also by Ingrid Clayton

Recovering Spirituality:
Achieving Emotional Sobriety
in your Spiritual Practice

Believing Me

**Healing from Narcissistic Abuse
and Complex Trauma**

A Memoir

Ingrid Clayton, PhD

My Own Voice Publishing

This book is a memoir and reflects the author's present recollections of experiences over time. Some names have been changed, some events have been compressed, and some dialogue has been recreated as truthfully as recollection permits.

The book is not intended to substitute for psychotherapy or professional advice. If you think you could benefit from therapy, contact a licensed mental health professional.

Printed in the United States of America.

For more information, or to book an event, contact:
www.IngridClayton.com

Author Photograph : Elaine Reid
Cover Design : Laura Shallcrass
Creative Consultant : Jillian Shillig

ISBN - Paperback: 979-8-9866187-0-8
ISBN - eBook: 979-8-9866187-1-5

First Edition: September, 2022

For my son, Henry.

And for her:

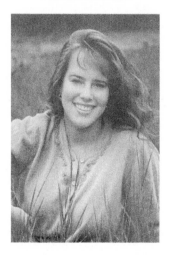

"Turn your pain into art."
— Claire Wineland

CONTENTS

Part Three: Trauma Healing

Prologue

Over the last thirty years, I have sought just about every imaginable remedy for the human condition. I've sat on therapists' couches to relieve my depression. I've meditated and practiced yoga to cope with anxiety. I've attended various twelve-step groups and have been clean and sober for over twenty-six years. I became a clinical psychologist, dedicating my life to helping other people heal. But in some ways, I remained unable to free myself from the past, bumping up against the same barriers: I don't know if what I think happened to me as a child actually did. And if it happened, was it that big of a deal?

I went on to specialize in trauma without fully recognizing the truth of my own. *Trauma* was a word reserved for people with a far "worse" story. Certainly a more visible one. Even when I became adept at recognizing my clients' experiences with relational trauma, how it manifested in a myriad of ways, I couldn't see myself that clearly. I could tell you the nuts and bolts of my story, but the impact was buried under decades of self-doubt.

Like most children, I started out with an uncensored and unashamed voice. Mine was largely a singing voice, belting out my sentences. I'd compose a showstopper about my grilled cheese, certain I was destined for Broadway by third grade. My first love was music and as I grew, so did my voice. It was bigger than anyone imagined such a tiny body could possess and wiser than my years on the planet.

I was a sponge, observing and analyzing everything going on around me. I trusted my gut and always knew my stepdad Randy was an arrogant bully, even though my mom adored him. He had this way of making other people think he was charming.

When Randy eventually crossed what seemed like obvious lines with me, I confided in my mom, but she didn't believe me. Randy called me a selfish liar—over the course of several years and with so much confidence—I wondered if it were true.

And so began the confusion of my truth, the loss of my voice. The constant downplaying of my experiences normalized the abnormal, becoming a blueprint for the way I saw myself and related to others. My self-hatred perpetuated and I began to compulsively seek healing, with little relief.

It wasn't until Randy's death in 2017, and the subsequent outing of other abusers during the #MeToo movement, that I began to find clarity, a reckoning with my history. I came to personally understand that trauma is less about a particular event and more about how we hold its effects in our nervous system, the way the experience lives on and defines the present moment. Trauma is the story we hold in the body.

This is the story I've been holding since I was thirteen and the puzzle pieces that finally allowed me to believe it. It's the story of redemption I never saw coming, in a manner I still find surprising. While I wasn't consciously pursuing healing, healing started pursuing me. After decades of trying to overcome my frailty, vulnerability, my madness—this is how I reclaimed my uncensored and unashamed voice. How I finally came to believe my own story, to believe myself.

***

If you happen to be reading this book because you found me on Instagram, know that this is the history and healing behind the open-hearted, humorous content I share there. It is not a textbook or how-to manual, but I have added a glossary of relevant terms and resources in the back of the book. While there are many ways to heal from trauma, if we can't see our narratives as traumatic, they are much harder to find. If people in the helping professions can't recognize trauma responses, they will continue to dismiss or misdiagnose them, further complicating access to proper support.

Validating my own experience was the turning point in my healing. Writing and sharing my story has provided more relief than anything else. If you see yourself reflected here, I hope it serves as validation for you. Your resonance and present-day symptoms are a bridge to healing. May you also come to believe yourself—love, advocate, find safety and relief for yourself, perhaps for the first time.

Part One: Traumatic Events

The Narcissist's Prayer

That didn't happen.
And if it did, it wasn't that bad.
And if it was, that's not a big deal.
And if it is, that's not my fault.
And if it was, I didn't mean it.
And if I did, you deserved it.

— Author Unknown

1

The Secret

Sometimes life and death happen so close to one another they appear interconnected. I married my husband Yancey in August, we bought a house in September, and I got pregnant with our son Henry in October. He was born just shy of my forty-first birthday.

In mid-April of 2016, Henry was nine months old and the perfect size for bathing in the kitchen sink at my cousin's flower farm in Colorado. My newly minted family was visiting my home state from Los Angeles, to introduce Henry to his relatives.

My mom had come down from the mountains earlier that week so she'd miss the storm. I thought my stepdad Randy would be with her, but he wasn't. Of course, I didn't want him there, but it still felt like a slap in the face when he made no effort to meet my son.

After Henry's fingers and toes were sufficiently nibbled by all, it was our last night in town. My mom pulled me aside. "I'd like to talk with you and Yancey in private after Henry goes to sleep," she said.

"Okay, is everything alright?"

"We'll just talk about it later," my mom said with her eyes closed, nodding her head in a directionless manner. She seemed so vulnerable, or maybe even angry, I couldn't tell. *Am I about to get in trouble?*

Yancey and I left the main house and tucked Henry in at the cottage house where we were sleeping. I grabbed a cozy blanket and sat cross-legged on the large, brown sectional in the living room. It was chilly and I wanted to warm up, but I was also attempting to mitigate what felt like a formal affair. It was unprecedented for my mom to summon me for a conversation.

She came into the room and sat a couple feet away from me. Yancey was sitting on the other wing of the couch. Before my mom said a word, she burst into tears.

"Oh, Mom!" I said. "What's going on?!" I gave her a hug, looking at Yancey with concern.

"I'm not supposed to tell anyone, so you can't say anything," my mom said, sobbing, "but I can't keep it a secret anymore. It's just too hard on me. Randy has lung cancer. He is dying and doesn't want anyone to know."

I sat there, stunned. Shocked.

My mom started speaking fast, as though she had to get the words out within a certain amount of time. "I'm terrified of being alone with him in that house, and that he'll take a long time to die. I just can't do it by myself. I don't know what I'll do if he hangs on for months and months."

I couldn't believe what she was saying. My shock had a numbing effect and I was trying to parse out what I was hearing. *Randy is dying.* My mom was obviously terrified, and yet I couldn't ignore the feelings that were bubbling up in me.

I had thought about Randy dying my entire life. I had fantasies in childhood about his funeral, where I would say everything I had always wanted. Or, I imagined not attending his funeral, as though my absence would offend him. Sometimes I fantasized he never existed, wondering how it might have felt to live with such ease.

I was trying to stay focused on my mom and what she was saying, but when I turned my attention to her experience I could only think, *Maybe she can be free?* She was still so young, only sixty-five. My mom could still have a full life, she could be independent. And if she could reconnect with her own thoughts and feelings... *Maybe I can get her back?*

My thoughts were racing as quickly as my mom was speaking. *Stay present, Ingrid.* I began to hone in on the emotional content of what she was saying. It seemed she wasn't as sad about Randy dying as she was worried about the possibility of him hanging on. Her honesty was profound. She rarely spoke about him or their relationship in a less than positive light.

I couldn't really take it in. All my fantasies of Randy's death were just that, an escape into another world. I always had to come back to reality, where no matter where I lived or what I was doing, Randy was somehow a part of that equation. It was like he lived in my very own cells.

The next morning, I reassured my mom that we would keep her secret. I told her she was going to be okay no matter what happened, because she was stronger than she realized. I really believed that. We said our goodbyes and I made her promise to stay in touch with any updates.

Back home in L.A., I began to wonder if I would get a call from Randy. I sort of knew I wouldn't, but this was his last chance to make things right. To tell my mom what really happened and maybe even apologize. I still had some hope of vindication before he died. Maybe not a conscious hope, but somewhere inside of me, I thought: *Is this how it's all going to end? No closure at all?*

I waited for a phone call that never came.

It wasn't until eight months later that Randy started telling the rest of the family he had cancer, and once he did, he declined quickly. Chemo only made him feel worse and hospice came into their home. My mom told me that a hospital bed was parked in their small living room and Randy hardly got out of it.

I was on edge all the time. Little things with Henry would set me off and I had no patience. I was doing my best to show up for my mom, checking in to see how she was coping or if there was any news. It was a lot, and I was overwhelmed.

"Hi, Mom, how are you?" I asked when I called.

Her voice always sounded like she wasn't in her body, as though I had asked her for a recipe. So, we didn't talk about feelings, just practical things. There was so much she didn't know how to navigate, because Randy had always handled the details.

"Don't worry," I said. "Henry and I will come visit and you won't be alone. We'll figure it all out together."

I meant that we would go *after* Randy died and thought this was clear. I had no intention of speaking with, or seeing him, at this point. He wasn't righting any wrongs, and I wasn't going to pretend none of it happened for one minute longer. This was a huge step for me. I had tolerated his presence long enough and I couldn't do it anymore.

The hospice nurse told my mom she was certain Randy would pass away in the next day or two, so I made travel plans for the following week. But then he had an energetic rally people often do at the end of their lives. He was hanging on and it was making me nervous.

It was one thing to say I'd go to Colorado *after* he passed away. It was another to tell my mom that we *weren't* coming in a few days if he were still alive. I was barely able to hold my newfound boundaries, I didn't feel like I could do it so intentionally, *out loud.*

I kept checking in a couple times a day. On one of our calls, I heard Randy in the background for the first time. His voice was gravelly and weak, but the same one that had haunted me since I was a kid. I could hear his words through the receiver, "Tell her I'm so happy they are coming."

Panic filled my veins and I became sick to my stomach. *He thinks I'm rushing to his bedside to pay my respects and introduce him to my son? NO!*

My mom started crying as though this was a sweet moment for us all. "Did you hear him, Ingrid? He's so happy you guys are coming," she said.

I was angry Randy knew we were coming, but even angrier my mom imagined this was a heart-warming situation. Fury rose from within.

"Yes, I heard him," I said. I tried to say it in a neutral tone. The straitjacket of my childhood was tightening under my skin, and before I suffocated, I had to get off the phone. "I have to run now, Mom. I'll call you later, okay?"

"What the FUCK?!" I yelled out loud in my kitchen. I knew I had to unequivocally let my mom know I would not be coming until after Randy died. *How could she expect me to come when he was still alive?* I knew I couldn't do it, but I felt so ashamed.

Don't good daughters support their mothers when a partner is dying? That seemed like the "right" thing to do. This was the first time in my life I knew how to minimize my feelings, but I couldn't imagine doing it. And the idea that Randy would be given any sort of grandfatherly title around Henry made me physically shake.

I gathered myself and called my sponsor, Bill. "How can I be such a cold-hearted daughter and not help my mom? What are people going to think? If I change plane tickets to avoid him, it seems so cruel!" I sobbed. "But I can't watch as he leaves this earth with all his secrets and lies!"

I told Bill how my cousins Megan and Erin had recently gone to the mountains, to support my mom. They assured me that even on his deathbed, Randy was reigning with terror. One night, he dragged his body from the hospital bed to get his laptop. When he saw my mom had learned how to pay their bills online, he became enraged, "What the fuck are you doing, Lynn?!" He was berating her for paying things out of his preferred sequence.

Bill heard everything I said and then asked me a simple question: "What would you do if you were putting yourself first in your own life?"

Gut punch. Deep breath.

My answer was obvious. If I were putting myself first, I would never see that man again and I would never subject Henry to his madness. The choice seemed clear, but I was still wavering. The stakes felt so high. The last time I took a real stand against my mom and Randy, I got burned. It made things worse. My entire body recoiled at the thought of standing up for myself again. Besides, my mom was in *distress!* Was now really the time to take care of *myself?*

After that phone call with Bill, I became willing to change our tickets, but I soon learned I didn't have to. My cousin texted: "He's gone."

Randy had drawn his last breath.

I was all alone in my living room when I heard the news. As I digested the fact of his passing, I began dropping deeper into my body than I had ever experienced. I thought, *This is not what you're supposed to feel when someone dies.* It wasn't the relief I had heard others express when someone's no longer suffering. I wasn't relieved for *him* that he was out of pain. I was alleviated of a heavy burden I had been carrying for over thirty years.

My therapist-self always wanted to believe the notion that if we forgive, we can be free. The reality is that I never had that experience. None of the "work" I had done on myself ever put a dent in the impact Randy made on me like his death was doing in that moment. I literally felt safer in the world knowing he was gone.

A knot I hadn't known was in my chest began to loosen and as I lingered in the space that was created, I observed a sense of freedom from within. I laid down on my hardwood floor and put my hand on my heart, like I was sandwiched between the earth and grace. I closed my eyes and let the truth of his passing wash over me. The truth of how it felt in my body as the straitjacket began melting into the floor. Then I knew I had to call my mom.

The very next day, Henry and I got on a plane. It was an enormous undertaking, but I didn't know I was about to go on an even bigger journey. One that took me back to the childhood I tried so hard to leave behind. Free from Randy's distortions and from the safety of my new life, I was about to become a witness to everything that happened and all the ways it shaped me. I was going to confront the past, even though my mom and Randy never did.

2

The Hot Tub

The Colorado sky was deep and vast at night. At thirteen years old, I loved sitting in the hot tub in the evenings with the lights from the house turned off so I could identify the constellations above. It was as though the stars reached into the water next to me and we reveled in the magic of the moment together.

The gurgling of the Roaring Fork River, as it carved its way through the Rockies, lulled me deeper into my own skin. In the winter, the snowdrifts came to the edge of the deck surrounding the sunken tub, and if I were feeling brave, I'd jump into the icy fluff. Barely able to catch my breath, my heart pulsing in my red, baby-faced cheeks, I'd quickly hop back to the safety of the cauldron and my extremities would tingle in excitement from the shock.

One night, my stepdad Randy came to join me in the hot tub. His legs were like tree trunks stomping on the deck, commanding all my attention. His shorts fit snug around the middle of his round belly where he carried an extra fifty pounds. Even in the winter, Randy always wore shorts. He'd tuck a tight-fitting t-shirt into his elastic waistband and proudly display a mariner's cross necklace on top. With his perm and full beard, my friends and I thought he looked like Captain Lou Albano, the professional wrestler.

I watched as he stepped into the tub, his trunks puffing up with air before sinking into the darkness below. Then I went back to star gazing, wondering which version of him I was getting: the one who seemed to despise me while correcting my every move, or the guy who thought he was likeable and kind. We sat in silence for a bit and then he started teasing me in a playful way.

"I bet you wish you could live up there with the stars, huh?" He laughed a little, but he wasn't laughing *at* me. It was like he was saying, *I know you wish you weren't here—with me—and that's okay.* It also felt like a nod to our shared passion, music. He knew I wanted to *be* a star, and when he heard me sing, a part of him thought I could.

There was no anger in his voice that night. It felt like he wanted to be my friend and I was relieved. I could feel my hard shell beginning to soften against the jets. I giggled as I wiped the blue eyeliner from under my eyes and started poking at my braces with my tongue. I hated the way my mouth looked but tried compensating with Silver City lipstick, the pink shade that was always sold out at the drug store. I thought it went well with the "blonde" streaks I'd added to my hair. I couldn't see it at the time, but no matter how much Sun In one used, brown hair only turned orange.

After another few moments of silence, Randy said, "Why don't you come sit on my lap, so you don't have to crank your neck?" He motioned that I could rest my head against his shoulder while looking up and I perceived it as an olive branch of stepfatherly love.

I went to his side of the tub and rested the back of my head against his chest. My legs were floating out in front of me while his arms anchored me in the water. I felt tethered, seen, and appreciated. It was a nice moment. The last three years had been so hard. Randy had moved in with my mom, brother Josh, and I almost as swiftly as our dad moved out. And then Randy kept moving us farther and farther away from our family and friends.

We'd been in Aspen for just over a year, and I still didn't seem to fit in. I felt like a city mouse and was missing my old life in Denver. Oddly, I felt like I was missing my mom too. It was like I'd watched her small frame slip directly into Randy's shadow. Her limbs only moved when his did, her words formed only when she'd heard him say them before. I felt like I was constantly wondering where my mom was, even when we stood in the same room.

Sitting in the hot tub, Randy began to squeeze my belly, just above my hips. "I like being this close to you," he said. "I'm so glad you don't seem to mind."

My thoughts began racing. *Why would he say that? Why would I mind? Is he implying I should mind, that maybe this is inappropriate?*

I didn't want to embarrass him (or me), and I didn't want to get in trouble for making the wrong assumption, so I asked him carefully, indirectly, with a neutral voice: "What do you mean, why would I mind?"

As I waited for his response, the prickliness of his body hair felt like needles on my skin. The water in the tub had created a suction between us and his fingers were like vice grips on my hips. I felt trapped as I held my body as still as possible.

"Some girls are uptight," he said. "They might want more personal space from the men in their lives." He paused and then continued. "I'm glad you aren't like them and that we can be this close."

That moment changed everything. At least it changed something in me. I was used to him being an asshole and I knew where I stood when he was yelling at me. I also knew when he was in a good mood, how he treated me when I was singing while he played piano. But this was different. His energy had changed, and rather than feeling taken care of, I felt terrified. I knew in my gut this wasn't right, but he was blurring boundaries in a seemingly harmless way, acting like nothing was wrong, and it paralyzed me.

I knew I couldn't trust him, but I couldn't trust my intuition in that situation either. I didn't know what seduction was—and wouldn't have the capacity to process the truth of that moment for many decades—but my body was clocking every second of the impact.

What I understood at the time was that if I followed his cues, I could likely maintain his affection and I wouldn't make things worse. I didn't feel safe, but I had to pretend otherwise. So, I lingered in the hot tub just long enough before saying I was ready to get out. I peeled myself off of his lap and wished I could blink myself into my bedroom as I stepped onto the deck. I wanted to run but needed to appear normal, so every step felt like it was in slow motion. A half-naked, soaking-wet, slow motion parade.

Arriving at the sliding glass door, I wanted to shake it all off, like an animal after they've been spooked. But I couldn't shake it. It was like I swallowed it down and it got stuck somewhere in my chest. I wanted to rewind the tape, to go back to moments before when I thought he was parenting me in a compassionate way. When he wanted to be my friend and I had some hope things could be *better*. I wanted this whole nightmare to be over. I wished, more than ever, I really could live up with the stars instead of sinking deeper into some unfathomable mire with Randy.

3

The Conductor's Baton

Randy used to be my dad's best friend. That's how he came into our lives. I can see his face amongst many memories and photographs of my parents' parties when they were still married. I was surrounded by beer bottles and metal strainers that separated the marijuana seeds from the buds.

I remember sitting in a circle one afternoon, in between my mom, dad and several of their friends. Listening to the Eagles, we were spread out on our orange, shag carpet as they passed a water bong around the room. I loved watching the bubbles through the clear glass.

"Let the kids take a hit," one of them said as they passed the bong directly to me. The round shape fit perfectly in my eight-year-old hands. I placed my lips to the circular glass and started to inhale, which made the bowl light up like a tiny brush fire. It made me nervous so I quickly passed the bong to the person next

21

to me, who then passed it to Josh—two and a half years younger than I. Josh took such a deep inhale that he immediately started coughing. This seemed to alert the adults that getting the kids stoned wasn't a great idea.

When I was ten and my brother Josh was eight, my mom and dad sat us down to say they were splitting up. The four of us sobbed like we were grieving the loss of something we didn't have to. I thought my parents were happy, skinny dipping with their friends in pools throughout our suburban neighborhood. But we quickly sold my childhood home, with my perfect pale-yellow bedroom and huge backyard, and Josh and I moved to a tiny apartment with our mom and Randy on the other side of Denver.

My familiarity with Randy didn't bring any comfort, it just made me mad, like I knew he belonged to another family and was taking up too much space in mine. I felt protective of my dad. It seemed like Randy had swept in while my dad's drinking was becoming more problematic. Like Randy was promising my mom a bigger life than my dad would ever afford. I guess my mom liked the sound of that.

In the evenings, the phone would ring in our new apartment. "This is the Denver County Jail, you have a collect call from…"

"I accept!" I'd yell while holding the receiver out so both Josh and I could press our faces to it. Our dad had gone to jail for a DUI and we missed him terribly.

"What did you have for dinner?" Josh asked with his delightful dimples and blonde hair.

"Tonight, I had steak!" our dad replied, "And now we get to watch some TV before bed." Jail sounded so *civilized*, and somehow better than our current circumstance in this ugly, brown apartment. I worried my dad might actually like it there. Maybe he would never pull himself together enough to make things right, so we could be a family again.

Nothing in my new world made sense except another dance routine to "I Would Die For You." I had recently traded my Olivia Newton John legwarmers for a *Purple Rain* inspired jacket and imagined being wild and free at a Prince concert, expertly articulating the hand signals to "die 4 you."

I was working on a routine in our living room, sweaty from some tricky choreography, when I took a bathroom break and found spots of blood in my underwear. I wanted to hide them but was afraid they'd be discovered, and then I would be discovered too. I was embarrassed, even ashamed. I wasn't sure what I was supposed to do.

I walked out to the kitchen where my mom was standing in front of the open refrigerator looking happy and pretty. It was like the refrigerator light was coming from inside of her, casting a warm glow on her Italian skin and short brown hair. She was talking with Randy sitting at the small kitchen table a few feet away.

I positioned myself between them, my back to Randy, and started tapping my mom on the arm. "Can you come with me, please?" I half-whispered and half-mouthed the question.

She kept brushing me off, then practically yelled: "What is it, Ingrid? Just tell me now." I couldn't believe she wanted me to spell it out in front of *him*. I grunted and walked awkwardly back to the bathroom where I stuffed toilet paper in my underwear, waiting for what felt like days for my mom to join me.

She finally found me in my room and I showed her the evidence without saying a word. "It's okay," she said before going to her bathroom to grab some supplies. My mom came back with giant pads that were too long for my underwear and so thick I could barely walk. I imagined my brother would think I just had a horseback lesson and hoped he wouldn't notice me at all.

My parents' divorce became final a few months later, and almost without warning, a pastor showed up at our condo in Golden, Colorado, to marry my mom and Randy in our living room. We had moved again, still farther from the place I called home.

I don't recall any witnesses of the ceremony besides Josh and myself, and I never saw photographs from the event. I later learned it was a secret Randy initially kept from his three kids. My mom was marriage number three and I suddenly had two stepbrothers and one stepsister.

Randy's lying by omission was a constant and curious thing. It was like he needed control at any cost. I could practically see him standing above all of us with a conductor's baton, choosing which voices could be heard and when. If one section of his life was at a crescendo, the rest became irrelevant; they could have disappeared altogether.

Randy's eldest kids lived in New Mexico, a composition from his past, but his youngest son, John, lived in a small mountain town about thirty miles from Aspen, where we moved next—probably so Randy could reestablish harmony with his favorite son.

John moved in with us shortly after we got to Aspen. I was twelve, John was eleven, and Josh was ten. The three of us got along okay, especially if we were playing Super Mario Brothers, but it was painfully obvious that whatever the rules were for Josh and I, they did not apply to Randy's "baby." If we received a small allowance, John got whatever he wanted. If the three of us had chores, John could do the bare minimum while Josh and I carried the load.

When we tried talking to our mom about it, her face would twist as nonsensical words fell from her lips. "Well … yeah … I don't …" It was like she had lost the ability to speak or hold any authority as our parent.

Randy, though, seemed to double down on the authoritarian role. I was rarely allowed to leave the house. I never had the same freedoms as my friends and could be grounded for weeks for the smallest infraction.

"Ingrid, did you write this message?" Randy asked one afternoon. I initially thought he was going to thank me because I took extra care to fill out all the quadrants on the pink message pad.

"Yes," I replied.

"Come here and look at this. How am I supposed to know when this person called?" He was acting as though I'd purposefully left a gas burner on in the kitchen. I wanted to say, *You could just ask me now*, but I knew to keep my mouth shut.

The rules were arbitrary, based on his mood. No matter how hard I tried to follow them, it was impossible. New standards erupted on the spot. They weren't age-appropriate lessons, with instructions or guidance, they were benchmarks I was meant to know in advance. When I didn't, I was grounded.

Spending so much time at home, I was grateful that at least our house was an upgrade. Eight miles from Main Street in Aspen, Colorado, our Woody Creek home had two stories, a spiral staircase and a steam room that made me feel like we were rich. Josh and I had bedrooms downstairs, and John's was upstairs next to "the parents," the shorthand we all used for our mom and his dad.

The upstairs living room had space for all of Randy's musical equipment: a professional-grade microphone and stand, a large drum kit for John, at least two electric keyboards, huge speakers, and a sound system. Randy had been playing music ever since his mom woke him in the middle of the night to play accordion for her guests. He started a band in his teens and aspired to be a professional musician. Although he never had lasting success, he saw himself as a musician above all else.

Randy could sing and play for hours, often the same songs over and over. Every now and then, he would want me to join him. He recognized my flair for the blues and taught me several old Bonnie Raitt songs. Without a word, Randy would start to play *Guilty*— that was my invitation. I recall feeling annoyed at the summons, always on his terms, but equally pleased it was finally my turn to sing.

I adjusted the mic stand while my vision softened the hard edges of our living room into an expansive space that felt personal to me. I held the mic in my right hand and the cord in my left, then closed my eyes and sang.

> *Got some whiskey from a bar man,*
> *Got some cocaine from a friend*
> *I just had to keep on moving,*
> *Till I was back in your arms again*
>
> *Well I'm guilty, yeah I'm guilty,*
> *I'll be guilty for the rest of my life...*

The lyrics were too mature for most twelve-year-olds, but inside I felt much older. Randy seemed to know I could handle singing songs about husbands who were cheating and lonely nights. I appreciated the nod to my maturity.

When my voice was amplified, it not only filled our house, it filled me up with an undeniable presence. I felt insulated from my insecurities and like I knew what it meant to be an old soul. I began to devour all of Randy's Bonnie Raitt records, her powerful voice gliding over the slide guitar. She had guts and I wanted that sort of confidence. I could almost taste it in the middle of a song. In between songs, I felt anxious, awkward and confused. I didn't know what to say or how to say it. But when I was singing, I could be brilliant.

Randy introduced me to my musical heroes. He loved it when I sang and he thought I could be great. If there were no other points of connection between us, at least we could agree on that. But there was a shadow side to feeling so seen and powerful. Looking back now, Randy seemed to be pulling me out of an innocence I wasn't entirely ready to leave. I could feel how discovering my own voice was tethered to him, like he wanted to own that part of me, or was using it in a way I didn't understand but detested. And all of this was woven into a larger tapestry of mixed messages: Sometimes I was unworthy, sometimes I was special. Either way—I was his.

4

A Belly Full of Air

Right as I was discovering my singing voice, I was seeing how ineffective it was in the rest of my life. In eighth grade at Aspen Middle School, we were assigned our first research paper. My friends were writing about fun topics like snowboarding, but I researched something I really wanted to understand. The title of my paper was: *Alcoholism: The Family Disease*. My dad had remarried by this time and between both my biological parents and their new spouses, I was starting to see how the disease was rotting my entire family tree.

My teacher called me in to her office after our papers were graded. I sat down and she slowly slid mine across her desk, almost like a secret note she was passing. I noticed the red "A-" written on the top while she started whispering questions about whether or not the subject was personal.

I responded candidly and watched as she closed her eyes for longer than felt comfortable, slowly nodding her head. She indicated that she admired my bravery, the maturity I must have possessed to write such a topic. While that may have been true, I felt disappointed that her focus was on my resilience rather than my family. I didn't want praise for surviving, I wanted something to change. Neither of us had anything else to say, so I scooped up the paper and went to my next class.

Back at home, I continued researching my parents' drinking and drug use. I was hungry for answers, for evidence of the dysfunction that always lay just beneath a "normal" façade. I always knew where their drugs were hidden and felt compelled to find them when they had been moved—above the refrigerator in one of the small cupboards; tucked under the headboard of my mom and Randy's waterbed; in the back corner of my mom's closet. The location changed but they were always in a small, round basket with brown stripes.

I'd carefully remove the matching woven lid to find several film canisters, vials and baggies with various amounts of dried plants and powder. One time, I found a silver hoover vacuum that looked like it belonged in a doll house, which I later learned was used for snorting cocaine.

I felt like I needed to know and understand everything I could about my mom and Randy. My fact-finding missions seemed to quell my deep sense of vulnerability and they became a life-long coping mechanism: trying to control whatever I could when my life felt so out of control.

***

We lived half a mile from the Woody Creek Tavern, a restaurant and bar that became my parents' second home. My brothers and I were invited to join them at the bar for dinner sometimes and it initially seemed fun.

Randy would walk in first; he loved a grand entrance. The bartenders were his buddies and the regulars were his friends. They would offer him a seat at the bar, but he'd make a joke about actually sitting at a table that night. Randy flirted with the waitresses and they flirted right back. We'd eat dinner and eventually my brothers and I would want to go home long before our parents were ready.

Josh, John, and I were left to entertain ourselves, playing pool and drinking too many cokes while our parents made their way to the bar. The longer we stayed, the more we saw other families come and go, the harder we tried to convince our parents to leave.

If it was my turn to approach them, I'd likely become the butt of Randy's jokes. On more than one occasion, he pretended to be selling me to a strange man at the bar who happily played along. I hated the charade, but that only seemed to make it funnier to them. My mom sat there silently caressing her wine glass with a permanent half-smile, her eyes blearily focused on nothing. We wouldn't be leaving anytime soon.

I'd often hear Randy talking about his business at the bar, how he moved to Aspen to sell "empty boxes." He would laugh his hyena-laugh as though he'd never told the joke before. The packaging and shipping store my parents opened was in the process of moving a Saudi Royal into his new Aspen ranch. Randy spoke about the job as though *he* were royalty.

What he didn't say was that he couldn't have started his business without my mom's sister, Janel. My aunt lived with us for a while in the caretaker unit attached to our Woody Creek house. She and my parents were initially business partners, but Randy saw himself as the boss. He and my aunt started fighting a lot and my mom was stuck in the middle. Things escalated and the next thing I knew, there was a lot of yelling about what Janel was owed and she was moving back to Denver.

I was in the caretaker unit with her as she was packing up her things. Watching as she folded the pink, oversized sweater I'd borrowed on several occasions, including picture day at school.

For the short time she was there, I loved having my aunt next door. She felt like a bridge to my old life. Her presence gave me comfort and reminded me of Sunday football, when my family would go to my aunt and uncle's house in Denver. The adults all wore Bronco orange and blue while Josh and I played with our three older cousins. My mom and Janel would make lasagna or spaghetti with Italian sausage and we'd all eat together, joking about who made the best garlic bread.

I was sitting on Janel's couch, watching her tape up another box when I noticed she was crying. "Are you okay?" I asked.

"I'm so worried about your mom. She doesn't understand what she's gotten herself into," Janel said.

I assumed she meant the general way Randy treated my mom. One might think her full name was, "Goddammit, Lynn," because it was often prefaced that way.

"The other night, I heard a crash coming from your house and I ran over to the kitchen," Janel continued. "When I opened the door, I saw your mom sitting at the table by herself. There was a large, red stain on the wall where a wineglass had shattered behind her."

Janel said my mom was staring off into space, almost unaware of the shards of glass at her feet. I was scared hearing this story, but not surprised. Janel was confirming what I already knew: Randy was a scary person.

Janel told me she asked my mom what happened and my mom replied, "Nothing."

"We've got to get out of here, Lynn," Janel said. "Come back to Denver with me."

She told me that eventually my mom agreed, saying only, "Okay, I'll go," as she kept staring straight ahead.

My body began to flood with something like relief. Like coming inside on a snowy day and drinking a hot cup of cocoa, the warmth was filling my belly and running down my limbs. *I have a witness.* There was an adult who saw what I thought I was seeing: Randy was dangerous, manipulative, and not to be trusted, and Janel had convinced my mom to leave!

But Janel continued, "The next morning, your mom changed her mind. She told me, 'Randy said everything going wrong around here is your fault. I'm not going to leave, but it's probably best if you do.'"

All the comfort I had felt began to curdle. I couldn't believe my mom was so close to leaving and then blamed her sister for all of it. *Everything going wrong is your fault.* I was beginning to see that Randy was never in the wrong and anyone who challenged him was condemned. I shared my own fears with Janel, and even though I was just a middle schooler, we had a mutual understanding. We were both heartbroken and equally powerless to do anything about it. Except Janel was free to go.

She said she was sorry to leave Josh and me, but she couldn't stay and be a silent witness. She and my mom would go through long periods of no-contact in the years to come. It always made me sad that my mom chose Randy over her only sister. She chose him over her friends and any life outside of their relationship. We were becoming more and more isolated, in the middle of nowhere, with no one to see what was really going on.

When Janel left, things got worse. No matter how lightly we all tread in the house, Randy's temper would eventually flare. One night he came home drunk and angry. He picked a fight with Josh, grabbing him by the collar and holding him several feet above the ground, firmly against the wall. He was yelling inches from Josh's face and Josh didn't yell back, but you could see how angry and frightened he was. Eventually, Randy dropped him and the fight, walking back to his bedroom for the night. The next morning it was like none of it happened. The terror always faded into the background, like a mirage, until the next time.

My mom's bruises would come and go. One day she'd have a black eye and tell us she fell on the corner of the coffee table, or that Randy had thrown the TV remote and she wasn't able to catch it. I always thought she was lying, but I never witnessed him hitting her, so I never knew for sure.

He never hit me, or grabbed me by the shirt. I didn't have any bruises, just a constant belly of air, holding it in as long as I could. I must have shared some of this with friends at school, because one of their moms called social services. They made a plan for me to go to Ashley's after school one day, where I'd meet with a social worker. I told my parents I was doing a school project and asked if they could pick me up after work.

I was nervous about the secrecy but glad someone intervened. I knew our homelife wasn't like all of my friends'. But I also felt confused over how my mom and Randy acted like nothing was wrong. They were successful business owners and got mad if we ever complained, highlighting all the ways we were taken care of. How we had a nice house. We had plenty to eat and I got new school clothes. Those things were true, so I didn't really know if I had it that bad.

Ashley and her mom left me alone in their living room with the social worker that afternoon. It was a brightly lit space with windows all around. The sunshine had a hopeful effect and the woman's clipboard seemed to say she was taking me seriously. I felt like I was with an expert who could truly evaluate my case.

We were sitting really close to one another as she started asking me specific questions. "Have you ever been hit by your parents?"

"No," I replied.

"Have you witnessed violence in your home?" she continued.

"Sort of," I said while sharing the way Randy would grab my brothers and shove them against the wall.

"Have you seen your stepdad hit your mom?" She seemed determined to find evidence of physical violence and I didn't have much to report. I told her how afraid my brothers and I felt when our parents were at the bar, how we never knew what it would be like when they got home. I told her about the yelling and getting grounded for nothing and I tried to share my fears, but she wasn't interested.

"I understand what you're saying, but these things aren't reportable," she told me. "Emotional abuse is not something we can intervene on and I was told there was physical violence happening in the home."

It was helpful to hear the term, "emotional abuse." I had never heard it before, but it clicked and felt official. The rest of her comment made me feel like I was wasting her time. I tried to explain my mom's bruises, but she was already packing up her clipboard. The assessment was over.

It was crushing to have the hope of an adult stepping in, followed by a determination that it wasn't "bad enough" to help me. Just like my teacher. Just like my aunt. Now with the social worker. I felt ashamed, like Ashley and her mom would think I was a liar. I took the social worker's lack of response as evidence for my parents' side of the story. Tipping the truth in their direction: *Everything is perfectly fine. If you don't think so, something is wrong with you.*

The seeds of self-doubt were planted and starting to grow. Despite what I witnessed on a daily basis—the bullying, temper flare-ups, active addictions and more—the adults who were supposed to help protect me were turning a deaf ear to my cries, making me question the validity of my voice if it wasn't entertaining them.

5

Getting Comfortable with the Uncomfortable

Randy was a compulsive liar. He made up outrageous stories all the time, like how he had been sky diving hundreds of times. I always knew he was hiding behind the lies, and that no one would ever know the entire story.

One night, when my brothers and I were home alone, the phone rang.

"Is Ben Webber there?" said the voice on the other end. It was a man's voice with a forced rasp and tone of mystery, similar to ones my friends and I once used to make prank phone calls.

"I'm sorry, but you must have the wrong number," I replied.

"Is Beeeen Webbeeer there?" he asked me again, stretching out the name a bit longer.

"There is no one here…," I said before the voice interrupted, "How about Randy, is *he* there? You should ask *him* about Ben Webber." Then the receiver went dead.

I hung up the downstairs phone feeling a little scared, as though a stranger was watching me through the curtains. My mom and Randy were at the Tavern, so I had to wait to ask them about Ben Webber the next day.

We were sitting at the kitchen table the next morning when I told them about the call.

Randy half smirked with a little sigh and I saw him retreat into his head for a moment. I looked to my mom for a reaction, but she wouldn't give me eye contact, so I looked back at Randy. "Do you know who that is?"

"What else did he say?" Randy asked.

"That was it. He just asked for Ben Webber two times, in a creepy way, and then mentioned you by name."

"If that ever happens again, I want you to get me immediately," Randy said.

"Well I would have, but you weren't here. And then he just hung up. Do you know who was calling?" I asked again.

Randy said he didn't know who called but that Ben Webber was the name he used when he and John were "on the lam" in Florida.

"What does that mean?" I asked.

Randy explained, candidly and casually, that when John was four years old, he picked him up from preschool and they left the state. Randy assumed the name, "Ben Webber," and they lived in Florida for almost three years. He didn't say, "I stole John away from his mom," or, "I abducted my son." He said, "on the lam," like they were in a big budget caper movie. And he talked about it as though it had happened a lifetime ago, when in reality, they had returned from Florida only five years previously. I was suddenly remembering how he had disappeared from our lives for a while.

This sounded horrible. And Randy was sharing it proudly, like he saw himself as a hero, a father protecting his son from harm. But there was no mention of harm. It made no sense to me.

I couldn't wait to ask John. The next time we were alone, I brought it up and was shocked to hear his response. "I loved being in Florida with my dad. It was like we were on permanent vacation," John said. Everything felt like a game, apparently, even looking out for the cops. John was instructed to yell out, "Dad, the heat!" whenever he saw a police car. They backed into parking spaces in case they needed a speedy getaway and John remembered there was a gun in the glovebox.

I could not believe what I was hearing. This was not the reaction I expected.

"Didn't you miss your mom? I don't understand why he took you from her?" I asked.

"It's weird, but I don't remember missing her. We never even talked about my mom; it was just like she was ... gone. My dad didn't want to share custody and wanted me for himself, so we just left," John said.

John's loyalty to his dad was unshakable. I wondered if Randy could do anything to tarnish John's impression. And everything must have worked out in the end because here we were, living thirty minutes away from John's mom Teri, and he was happily going back and forth between homes.

I never found out who called for Ben Webber or why they were calling. And hearing the details about Florida didn't give me clarity as much as it created more questions. One of the biggest of which was why my mom chose to look the other way.

I knew that sometimes she caught glimpses of the Randy I saw. A couple of years after we had moved to Aspen, I was fourteen when I heard my mom sobbing in her bedroom. I ran in to find her collapsed on the bed. "I'm going to leave him," she said. "I don't know what we will do, but we have to go."

I practically jumped up and down. "Yes, yes! We can do this, Mom. I know we can!"

She kept saying, "I don't know what we will do," which I interpreted to mean we didn't have any money, but I tried to reassure her we'd figure it out.

"Should we pack some things and go right now?" I asked.

"No, not yet." She was still bawling. "Just give me some time."

"Okay, Mom. I love you. It's going to be okay," I said before leaving her bedroom. I walked into the living room and immediately felt like it wasn't mine. Like we were already gone. I populated my mind with fantasies of living in a small apartment with my mom and Josh. It was sparse, but we loved it because she was there. We had our mom back. I wouldn't have to worry about Randy's unpredictable moods or inappropriate gaze—both had me feeling like a sitting duck. I didn't care if we had to live in a shelter, as long as we were free.

I don't remember how long it was before we talked about it again, but by then my mom's sorrow had dissipated. It was almost like we never shared that moment in her bedroom. "No, we aren't going anywhere," she said, as though it were a silly idea.

I was crushed and couldn't comprehend her decision.

I recalled how she was crowned Miss Thornton in 1969. There was a blue and silver pageant trophy in our basement when I was a little girl. It was the same height as me and I would take the tiny scepter out of the tiny women's hand atop the glittery prize and march around with it like I was in a parade. I loved the black and white photos of my mom with a satin sash and up-do, smiling for the papers. She looked truly happy, truly alive.

I wanted so much to be like her when I grew up, but I didn't feel that way anymore. That version of her seemed gone. The confidence she once possessed had disappeared. Even when she was around, she was always in the background.

***

Like so many frightening events involving Randy, my mom was absent the night he drove my brothers and I over Watson Divide Road. It was a shortcut to our new house in Old Snowmass, an even more remote town than Woody Creek, fifteen miles northwest of Aspen.

The road itself was gravel and no matter how often it had been groomed, there were always large pits and accordion-like patches that vibrated your soul as the wheels rolled over. Watsons was narrow and winding, best fit for one car even though people drove it in both directions, and it had no guardrails.

I was fifteen on this night and digging my nails into the door handle. Randy was so drunk he couldn't stay centered on the road. Several times he got dangerously close to the steep cliff before jerking back towards the hillside. It was dark and I watched as our headlights bobbed and weaved around our certain death. I'm sure my brothers were silently praying with me: *Please, God, help us make it home.*

We eventually made it off the dirt road and onto the paved one leading to our small cul-de-sac. As Randy pulled into our driveway and put the minivan in park, John started yelling. "That was really messed up, Dad! You could have killed us!"

Randy grabbed the boxes of pizza that were meant for dinner and hurled them all over the yard. Slices went flying as he screamed at all three of us, "How dare you question my authority!" He yelled at us to go inside and we all went to our rooms without dinner.

The next morning, Randy called us into the kitchen. We gathered around the sink and I noticed several bottles of booze on the counter, the large ones with the big handle. "I want you to watch me pour every drop down the drain," he said as he turned the vodka bottle upside down.

Then he proceeded to make a dramatic speech, the theme of which was, "It takes a big person to see the error of his ways."

Instead of apologizing for what happened the night before, he expected us to applaud this grand gesture. I watched, disgusted, as John gave him praise. "Good job, Dad. I'm proud of you."

It all seemed like a charade. Randy wasn't remorseful and he was jumping to the part of the story where everyone was supposed to be grateful. It made me sick, but I complied with the theatrics. "That's great. Good for you." I didn't mean a word.

Weeks later, we were sitting in a restaurant for Mother's Day brunch when Randy ordered mimosas. I was furious and said from across the table, "Did you jump off the wagon?"

He cleared his throat and licked his lips, shooting an angry glare in my direction. "The expression is *falling* off the wagon," he said.

"Yeah, I know what the expression is," I said, thinking my verb choice had made my case. That was the end of the discussion. We never addressed his pledge of abstinence again.

We continued to enjoy a pleasant Mother's Day morning, celebrating my mom by watching them drink mimosas. In some ways this was fine by my brothers and me. Who doesn't want to enjoy eggs benedict at a fancy restaurant rather than feeling betrayal? Numbness was easier. Going along with the happy family charade was simpler. Calling out Randy's behavior meant bearing the brunt of his anger and hostility. As I cozied up to denial, perhaps I understood my mom more than I realized. Maybe I was growing up to be like her after all.

6

The Wrecking Ball

If you asked most teenagers what they wanted in life, I doubt they would have said, "something boring, predictable, *normal.*" But that's all I ever wanted, and life with Randy was anything but. It was a pendulum swinging between two extremes: being painfully ignored by him or being the focus of his not-so-fatherly attention. I never knew what Randy's mood would be, and it was safer just to get out of his way.

Many nights in Old Snowmass my brothers and I would heat up a Hot Pocket and watch TV while our parents were at the Tavern. They kept their allegiance to the bar, even though the commute went from two minutes to twenty.

We knew the Tavern's phone number by heart and the bartenders recognized all of our voices. We'd often call to find out when our parents would be home, hours after they said they'd be.

"It's your kids," we'd hear one of the bartenders laugh, "you're busted!" And then they passed the phone to Randy—always to Randy—never to my mom.

Eventually, we saw headlights flash on our detached garage and heard tires coming down the gravel driveway. My stomach dropped and without talking to one another, my brothers and I scrambled to turn off the TV and ran to our rooms.

On many of those nights, I heard Randy come back towards my bedroom, because it was right next to John's room. John and I were on one side of the house, our parents on the other, while Josh lived in the middle ground, tucked up above the living room in a small, open loft.

I would hear Randy through my thin bedroom walls, "Hey, bud ..." expressing affection and curiosity about John's day. Hearing such loving attention felt like a twist of the knife. It was bad enough we all ran to our rooms, but only one of us was sought after. I never wanted Randy to knock on my door, but I wondered if my mom was ever curious about my day. If she would ever come to my room just to tell me she loved me.

Months would go by where I was simply ignored in our home, like I didn't exist. My brothers and I would be eating breakfast at the kitchen table when Randy came in. "Good morning, John. Good morning, Josh," he'd gush, like we were The Waltons, but there was no greeting for me.

The same thing happened when he dropped us off at school. "Have a good day, pal," he'd say to Josh at the middle school. Then at the high school, "I love you, buddy," to John. I would exit the minivan in silence, feeling the heat of Randy's hatred on my back as I walked away. He never even looked in my direction as he waited for the sliding door of the van to close behind me.

I didn't know why he gave me the silent treatment. I strained to not let it bother me, but it really did. *Was it because I talked back? Was it because he knew I didn't like him?* I certainly wasn't an angel, but I couldn't understand his behavior.

Morning after morning, I'd sit behind Randy and John for our forty-five-minute commute to school, feeling like the evil stepdaughter, a forced witness to their love. It wasn't just a sweet connection between father and son, it felt like a conversation "at" me. Randy was being a bully by excluding me in a specific way. His admiration and cheerleading of John was letting me know it was possible, but not for me. Josh didn't seem bothered, but he wasn't ignored.

I struggled to hide my hurt as I walked onto campus, but there were days when it was impossible. One morning in particular, I ducked into the girl's locker room on the first floor to get a hold of myself. I walked over to the mirror and felt the weight of my body prop against the small porcelain sink. I was looking for answers in my reflected face, but when I only saw sadness, I backed up against the painted cinder blocks, "Aspen Skiers," and slid down to the cold, cement floor, where I started to cry.

My tears had sound that echoed against the metal and concrete. Part of me wanted someone to come in, to see me in the pain of that moment. But no one came. Eventually my sadness shifted to self-consciousness. I was certain I'd be labeled an attention-seeking loser if anyone were to find me there.

I stood up and once again looked in the mirror. "Get it together, Ingrid," I mouthed to myself. I had to tuck my defeat into one of the lockers that surrounded me so I could ascend the stairs and greet my friends with a smile on my face.

***

It was easy to hate Randy for ignoring me, because I could see myself strictly as a victim. It was harder to understand my feelings when he stopped. It awakened a part of me that desperately needed to be seen. I would find myself "forgiving" his abuses in exchange for moments of his favor. Even then, I was aware that it came at a price, but it was monumentally preferable to feeling invisible and despised.

One day, Randy asked if he could pick me up from school to take me to lunch. The invitation was surprising. He was seething at me the day before, and now we had a lunch date.

Knowing how much I loved Italian food, he was taking me to a new wood-fire Italian Restaurant called Mezzaluna on Cooper Street in Aspen. I suddenly felt special: my chest opened up, allowing me to breathe a little deeper.

As we left my school and drove into town, Randy was inquisitive, like he needed to catch up on everything he had missed in the months prior. I was sitting in the front seat for a change and noticed I was shaking as we crossed Castle Creek Bridge. It wasn't the temperature or how high we were suspended above ground; it was raw nerves exposing my apprehension. The shift from icing me out to shining such a glow was disorienting.

Walking into the restaurant, I felt the heat from the wood burning fire and smelled a mixture of fresh dough, olive oil and roasted garlic—my version of heaven. The maî·tre d' asked Randy where he'd like to sit. "How about there?" He pointed to what looked like the best seat in the house.

I attempted to sit a little taller at the table, hoping to look as though this lunch was an everyday occurrence. Like it was no big deal to be pampered and to feel alive in Randy's presence. A part of me didn't want to give him the satisfaction, but most of me didn't care because it felt so good.

I felt my rage slipping away at the table-for-two in the window. The sun warmed my face as we chatted over fresh bread. I felt like I'd stepped out of a black and white version of myself and into full, vibrant color.

Having Randy's undivided attention gave me a sense of power that was both confusing and intoxicating. I knew I could get whatever I wanted and was going to take full advantage of it. I would be pleasing, doting, and ever lovely for the remainder of the meal and for however long his affection might last. I was aware he didn't invite my mom to lunch, and imagined she didn't even know about it—a detail that remained just below conscious awareness as I devoured my ravioli.

When we finished eating, Randy noticed Chepita, the jewelry store across the street. He said he had some business to do there, and I excitedly accommodated his request to stop by the store, thinking I'd browse while they talked about boxes and gift bags.

There was a ring I had been coveting in the display case. My best friend Mita and I would often see it in the window, and I'd even gone in to try it on. Randy started chatting up the saleswoman and when there was a lull in their conversation, I called him over to the display, loud enough for the woman to hear. "Randy, come here. You've got to see this gorgeous ring. I haven't been able to stop thinking about it."

It was twenty-four karat gold with two pink tourmaline, pear-shaped stones and tiny diamonds flanking both sides. It was pricey, but I could see Randy playing the big shot for the saleswoman, who also knew how to play up displays of affection. The three of us began to whip up such a frenzy about his generosity, the beauty of the ring, what a lucky girl I was … there was no other ending to the story but me walking away with the ring.

The saleswoman put it in a beautiful box and bag before holding it out in front of her, querying who she should pass it to. Randy stepped aside and gestured towards me, "You can give it to Her Highness."

I reached for the bag and looked the woman in the eyes. "Thank you so much," I said, hoping my gratitude aimed at her was enough to satisfy Randy. Then he and I walked outside. "Can I put it on now?" I asked.

"Of course," he said.

Standing in front of the store, I put the ring on my left ring finger, where it fit perfectly. I couldn't stop staring at my hand. I stretched my arm out in the sun and watched how the stones glistened.

"Isn't it incredible?" I asked Randy.

"Yeah," he said, somewhat truncated and in a lower register than before and I immediately wondered if he had buyer's remorse. The enthusiasm he had demonstrated moments before was gone.

I profusely thanked him for his generosity, not just because it was true, but because I wanted to reignite his spark.

"You're welcome," he said. "I've gotta get back to the office. Let's hit the road."

We walked towards the car and with every step, something was starting to stir behind my triumph. Anxiety was blurring my appreciation. A part of me felt like I'd just made a deal with the devil.

It may have appeared to others like a father and daughter out for a lovely lunch. I certainly gave off that appearance. I was like a robot, knowing when to laugh and when to compliment. When to give Randy the praise I knew he needed.

But behind that façade, I felt dirty. Like I was selling my integrity to get some love and attention, to get a beautiful ring. Like I was letting Randy off the hook for the ways he intentionally squashed my spirit. Accepting the ring felt like absolution; even prostitution. The feeling in my body was one of repulsion. There was no self-esteem tucked inside those mechanics. No self at all.

As we reached the minivan, my complicated internal world became even more crowded. I wondered what my mom would think if she were there. I suspected I would not be wearing the ring. He wouldn't have bought me such a gift in her presence. I projected this thought onto Randy's urgency to leave, imagining he was already minimizing the jewelry and lunch date in anticipation of seeing my mom back at their store.

I could feel in that moment how my mom and I were on opposite ends of Randy's world, our relationship obscured by the wrecking ball between us.

My mom couldn't see me, or even know me, because Randy was always in the way, threatening, intimidating, and keeping the two of us from ever getting close.

She didn't take me to lunch that day, or any other. She didn't seek out one-on-one time and I knew it wasn't really a possibility. If she had, she might have seen the position I was in. How I was maneuvering through the madness of Randy's mood swings and hating myself for it. She might have seen how she was doing the same. But he would never let that happen.

7

The Invitation

With no warning, my mom left for Texas. Her parents were travelling cross-country in their motorhome when my grandfather became too ill to drive. We soon learned he was dying of cancer and they needed my mom's help. She never travelled alone, but she quickly packed her things and prepared to be gone for some time.

Not long after my mom left, Randy came back to my room one night. I was irritated to see him standing there and assumed I was about to get in trouble. We were back in a long stretch of detesting one another.

"How's it going?" he asked as he filled the entire doorframe.

I started fiddling with my ring. I wore it every day and would often rotate it in this compulsive manner. I still loved it, even though Randy and I never spoke of it again. When my mom saw it for the first time, she couldn't easily hide her disapproval, but she couldn't voice it either.

I twirled the ring around one more time as I waited to see if he had more to say, then said, "I'm fine."

"Hey, how'd you like to go to Las Vegas?" he asked.

"What?" I was truly confused.

"Obviously as a singer, you would want to witness that sort of professionalism," he replied. "There are incredible shows with real entertainers in Vegas. It would be great for you to see how things are really done."

"Sure, I'd like to go to Vegas one day," I said, hunching my shoulders to express the implausibility. I had often dreamt about life in New York, Los Angeles, and sure … Las Vegas would be interesting.

"Well, let's go," he replied.

"What do you mean?" I was completely caught off guard.

"Pack a bag for a few days and hide it in your closet. I'll drop you guys off at school like usual, but then I'll come back to grab our luggage when the boys aren't in the car," he said.

I felt frozen. *He wants me to go to Las Vegas with him this weekend?* The way he presented the trip made me feel like a refusal would be saying "no" to my dreams. I kept staring in silence.

"Listen, it's no big deal. I was given a couple of tickets to Vegas and since your mom isn't around, I thought it would be fun to take you. But if you don't want to go, I'll take John."

I still couldn't comprehend what was happening, but I didn't want him to take the opportunity away. "I want to go," I said. "I just don't know why it's a secret from the boys."

"I can't take everyone and I don't want them to be jealous. I made arrangements for John to stay with his mom, and Josh to stay with friends. They think you'll be at Mita's house and that I'm going out of town on business."

I felt uneasy about the secrecy, but it seemed like Randy had already told the boys his lie. It was a fast-moving train and the rapid shift from adversary to protégé was a welcomed one. I had quick flashes of who I might meet on the Las Vegas Strip. I imagined being "discovered" in a casino, as though music producers were hiding behind slot machines just waiting to award the biggest jackpot of all: "Ingrid Bollman, you are the star we've been waiting for!"

"Okay, let's go," I said. "What do I need to pack?"

Randy had this look on his face, like he knew he had me in the palm of his hand. He was adoring me and I was adoring that feeling. It was alchemical. We were about to go on an adventure.

"Don't worry about it too much. We can buy some things when we get to town. Just let me handle the details." And then he walked back to his bedroom on the other side of the house.

It happened so quickly, I almost felt like we had planned the getaway together. I closed my bedroom door and started looking in my closet, pulling dresses off of hangers and grabbing my favorite jeans.

When my bag was packed, I put it in my closet, then went to sit on my bed. I felt like static electricity was running through me and it was hard to finish a thought. I brushed my teeth, hoping the nighttime routine would lull me into exhaustion, but I was still wired as I lay back on my bed.

I went back to my desk, where I'd been sitting when Randy came to my room. I quietly picked up the receiver on my Mickey Mouse phone and dialed Randy's oldest son, Sean.

Sean was six years older than me and he'd been living down the road from us in Old Snowmass for about a year. He had come back into Randy's life and worked for him at the packaging and shipping store. Sean and I could be honest with each other. I never had to sugarcoat my feelings about his dad and he didn't sugarcoat things either.

Sean once told me Randy had said inappropriate things about me, talking about my body in a sexual way. I felt disgusted, but was grateful Sean was honest, and that he responded to his dad by saying, "Jesus, don't talk about Ingrid that way!"

I somehow imagined that all stepdaughters must find themselves in this situation when they go through puberty. *How hard must it be for a man who isn't blood related, to see his stepdaughter as something other than a sex object?* I think I was trying to normalize what felt like such an assault.

"Hello," Sean said before I responded in a whisper.

"No one else knows about this." I was pressing my ear against the phone, making sure Randy didn't pick up the line in the other room.

"What's going on, Fea?" Sean always called me "ugly girl" in Spanish. I hated it, but he had been doing it so long, the word almost lost all meaning.

"Your dad wants to take me to Vegas this weekend and to keep it a secret from Josh and John."

"What? That motherfucker," Sean said. I could hear people in the background. There was music and laughter, and Sean told them to keep it down.

"I know. It's kind of crazy and I'm not sure what to do." I wanted Sean to fix it somehow. Not in a confrontational way. That felt scarier than the situation I was in. I wanted him to fix it in a *magical* kind of way. Maybe if Sean saw this as an exciting trip, I could actually believe it.

"I think I should just go, and hope it's the trip he's promising ... seeing some shows and getting musical inspiration. But I need someone to know where I am, or something to do in case it gets weird. I don't really know what could happen."

Sean was relaying what I was saying to his girlfriend and their friends. I felt comforted by the fact that they were all suddenly quiet, taking this seriously, and helping me figure out a plan.

"I think you're right not to make waves in advance," Sean said. "Whatever you try, no one will listen. The old man will make up some bullshit story and get away with it like always. Then it will backfire on you," he said.

Sinking deeper onto my desk, I knew he was right. One of Randy's favorite sayings was, "If you throw enough bullshit against the wall, some of it is going to stick." His confidence was like hypnosis. And as much as Randy had the power to give me the world, he could lock me away from it with no remorse. It felt like a no-win situation to disrupt the plan in advance.

"So, I should just go and hope it's a fun trip?" I asked.

Neither of us were acknowledging Randy's capacity to sexualize me, or that I could be in any real danger. I was *feeling* like I could be in danger, and I suspect he was too, but we didn't say that out loud.

It was fucked up that Randy was lying to the boys, that part was obvious. But maybe there was nothing else nefarious going on? Maybe he really didn't want to deal with the jealousy of choosing only one of us.

It was alluring to think I was being spoiled and my talents were worth such an investment. And even if this was a bigger deal than I'd ever experienced, it wasn't unheard of for Randy to surprise me with outrageous displays of affection.

I decided to go along with Randy's plan. Sean gave me the number of some friends who lived in Vegas. They said they'd make themselves available if I needed anything and Sean told me he would drive to Vegas to pick me up if he had to.

On Friday morning, Randy drove us to school like usual. John sat in the front while Josh and I rode in the back. Steely Dan was blaring and I was glad to have a soundtrack playing over my thoughts.

No one said much in the car. I didn't want to tip the boys off to what was about to happen and I wasn't sure if we would really go through with it. I stared out the window and compulsively chewed the inside of my cheek, hoping I wouldn't dig too far into the soft flesh.

We stopped at the middle school, and then the high school where John and I said our goodbyes to his dad. It was as though we both planned to see him on Sunday night. "Have a good weekend," we all said before Randy drove away, circling back home to get our luggage.

In the few hours before he returned to school, I broke my promise to keep the trip a secret again. "Dude, you aren't going to believe this," I said to Mita in front of our shared locker with our favorite BFF photos taped inside. "Randy is taking me to Las Vegas today."

I think I was looking for a certain reaction from Mita, too. I often felt like I was riding in her sidecar. She was the youngest of five sisters, all with a certain star quality. I liked to imagine I was sister number six, sort of the runt of the litter. That morning, I was feeling particularly scrawny and needed Mita's guidance.

"What's that all about?" Mita asked. I wasn't sure if I was reading jealousy or annoyance in her voice, but I could feel her emotional distance. It felt like I just told her I was going to do math homework.

"He wants to take me to see some professional shows," I said while thinking, *Randy and I are going alone.*

"Dude, that's crazy," Mita said. She brushed her long bangs away from her forehead and turned to look for our friends down the hall. She was ready to move on from our conversation so I left it at that. *Maybe I'm making something out of nothing.*

***

I met Randy in the front office around 10:00 a.m. and he told the school secretary I wouldn't be back for the rest of the day.

My heart raced as we drove away from the Maroon Bells, the protective peaks that watched over Aspen High. Randy seemed like a giddy teenager as we turned the corner onto Highway 82, towards the airport that sat directly across from the business center where he was playing hooky.

This was new territory, and I wasn't sure how to behave. The stakes felt higher than the jewelry store or when I was singing with him. I still wanted to maintain his affection, but I was strapped into a ride I had never been on and wasn't sure if I was going to like it.

I looked over at Randy while he laughed at his own joke, noticing his silver earrings and how long his hair had grown in the back. I saw the mole on the side of his neck, escaping like a worm, and decided to keep my eyes straight ahead for the rest of the drive.

I took a deep breath and chose to go along with the spirit of adventure. I wanted to believe this trip was for *me*. That he wanted to inspire me, and I deserved such care and attention. I started asking Randy questions about the last time he was in Vegas or if he had ever played music there. I was trying to get excited.

Arriving at the airport, it wasn't long before we boarded our plane. We were sitting in a two-seater row when Randy casually mentioned, "This trip is costing me a fortune, so I only got us one hotel room."

The sound of my pulse reverberated against the seatbelt. I became aware of just how tightly it was holding me in place. I remembered that night in the hot tub years ago, how the tone of his voice made the hair stand up on my neck. It was happening again. I interpreted him to mean, *I'm being very generous, don't push me on this*, as another boundary was being blurred. I also recalled how he said he got free tickets from a friend. "This trip is costing me a fortune," didn't match that story.

We took off and I heard the wheels lift off the runway, hiding neatly into the belly of the plane. My adrenaline gave me the courage to question all the secrecy. "This is a really amazing gift you're giving me, one that might be life changing. It seems strange I can't tell anyone about it." I was trying to appeal to his grandiose nature, wriggling my way out of what I later came to know as gaslighting—manipulating my perception until I questioned my own sanity.

He explained again that telling people would only make them jealous. He didn't want my brothers to feel bad, and he didn't want my mom to know we were off having fun while she was going through such a difficult time.

In that moment, it really hit me. *My mom doesn't know he's taking me away.* Maybe I knew it intuitively, but having it confirmed pierced the delusion. Of course, he was lying to her too. The gravity of my situation was getting clearer the higher we climbed.

He eventually gave in to my request for transparency. "I'll tell them, but you have to let me do it *my way*," he said before ordering his first vodka of the day. I wasn't sure what that meant, but I allowed it to calm my nerves. Stories from his past were flooding my consciousness and I was desperately trying to determine my place on the vulnerability scale.

A part of me was thinking about John, how he was taken to Florida for almost three years. Then I thought about his mom, Teri. I knew she was really young when she married Randy. I think he was cheating on his first wife and kids in order to be with her.

Hearing Randy would tell my mom about Vegas made me believe we had a round-trip ticket. It made me feel like he had at least one foot in reality, one foot in his marriage to my mom. Even if he was wooing her daughter, behind her back, he was still committed to that relationship in some way. I was growing terrified, but had to abandon my terror in favor of a more innocent version of the story. As I looked out the window, the spectacular mountain ranges below were being transformed into tiny anthills, shape shifting my reality by the second.

8

What Happens in Vegas

Arriving at the Tropicana was like stepping into a postcard. I almost wanted to poke the air to see if it had paper edges. Cigarette smoke filled the atmosphere and mixed with exhaust from the taxi as we retrieved our luggage from the trunk. Hundreds of light bulbs made up the entranceway, twinkling in the bright desert daylight. It was the first of many tricks the environment would play on my senses, and I began to wonder if it was day or night.

Standing at the front desk with Randy was awkward. I was sixteen, with long dark hair, full eyebrows, and a fair-skinned baby face. I loved it when people said I looked like Ione Skye, from *Say Anything* but in that moment, I knew I needed to play an *older* part. This was an unspoken expectation and I wasn't sure how to do it, so I just stood there with a fake smile on my face.

Neither of us spoke as we entered our faux Floridian suite. It was wrapped in bamboo and eighties-era textiles. To the right of the door was a giant king bed, not two queens like I was expecting. My eyes locked on the maroon and teal bedspread. It assaulted my senses with large blocks of color that seemed to be hiding an unsavory past. There was a mirrored headboard and— *What is going on, there is a mirror on the ceiling?!*

This detail set off alarm bells. I felt a paralysis, similar to when I first became aware of my body in puberty. I remembered lying on the couch at my dad's house when a commercial for tampons came on TV. I started to hold my breath from the sheer embarrassment of the moment. I hoped my stillness might allow me to disappear. I wanted the commercial to end, and for no one in the room to think of me in relation to it. That is how I felt in that hotel room: in desperate denial of my developing body, or rather a need to deny that anyone else could see it.

I continued to survey the room. At the far end were matching window treatments chintzily hanging like eyebrows above the loveseat and chairs. Smoke-stained fabric covered the cushions that were pilling from overuse. There was a glass ashtray on the coffee table.

"Did you bring your cigarettes?" Randy asked. I had never smoked in front of him but I figured he had probably seen a pack in my sock drawer. I knew he snooped through my things because months earlier he had yelled at me, "I know you think we're alcoholics who live at the bar," as though he were Svengali, reading my mind.

In truth, he was quoting an exact sentence I had written in my diary before all my journals went mysteriously missing. I couldn't believe he thought I wouldn't put it together. "Did you steal my journals?!" I yelled back.

He ignored me and stomped away. I never saw my cloth-covered notebooks again. Years of my inner life, containing bubble letters, school crushes, and my attempts to understand and survive my home life… all stolen.

Now he was letting me know that he knew my secret and was inviting that part of me into this fantastical world. But I had no intention of smoking in front of him. In another scenario, he would use my habit as a way to ground me for a semester. He may have sleuthed his way into getting more information, but I wasn't going to hand over my private life so freely.

I gave a little laugh at his question and said, "No," leaving it at that.

As we started to unpack, Randy told me the plans for the rest of the day. First, we had to get me some new clothes. He wanted me to appear more "sophisticated."

"Casinos don't allow minors, so people need to think we're together or you'll get kicked out and I'll get in trouble. You also need to hold my hand everywhere we go," he said.

The teenage girl in me welcomed the shopping spree and I immediately minimized the rest. I knew he was lying—but wasn't sure which parts were a lie. *Did casinos allow minors? Could we get in trouble?* The only thing I knew for sure was I could get in trouble with *him.*

As we approached the main casino for the first time, Randy grabbed my hand. It didn't gross me out like I thought it might. It had the effect of elevating my status somehow. Like I was actually older in that moment, more mature and deserving of respect. I looked down row after row of noisy slot machines.

"Do you wanna play?" Randy asked.

"Can I?"

"Well, let me do it for you." He grabbed a wad of hundred-dollar-bills from his pocket, removing the silver money clip as he told me to choose a machine. I chose a quarter slot machine with red flames surrounding it. Randy and I looked around and didn't see anyone close by. He put the money in and said, "pull the lever."

I grabbed the knob on the side of the machine and the wheels started spinning. As each one came to a stop, I waited for the coins to fall into the tray, but nothing happened. "Oh man," I said. "That was disappointing."

I felt Randy watching me, as though my reaction was his entertainment. We pulled the lever several more times, to the same outcome. "Let's go shopping," he said.

The first outfit I chose was a chocolate brown blazer and matching silk shorts. The blazer had amazing shoulder pads and paired perfectly with a cream, silk shirt. The ensemble made me feel more "put together" then I ever had, and the abundance had a dizzying effect. *Jackpot.*

With my giant Banana Republic bag in tow, we continued to several more stores. Walking by a Benetton, I looked up at Randy. I knew their clothes were expensive, but I scrunched my face and raised one shoulder as if to say, "You think we could go in?"

"Let's go," he said.

As I walked into the store, I could feel our distance from Aspen, from the rest of the family, and any reservations I might have had about being so spoiled. I loved that I could try anything on and eventually picked out a gorgeous wool sweater I couldn't wait to wear when we got home.

With my arms draped in shopping bags, we went back to the hotel and got dressed for the night. We had tickets to *Folies Bergère*, the famed "longest running show in the history of Vegas." Randy just needed to see some "old friends" first.

This was a surprising detail given all our duck and cover. I asked who we were meeting, but Randy kept it vague. "They're just some old friends from Florida," he said. This made me nervous, reconnecting the dots of our secret escape to the one he'd made with John.

We got in a cab and drove to the end of a strip mall fifteen minutes away. As we walked in the restaurant, Randy noticed his friends, a couple, sitting in the darkly lit room. We all said a quick "Hello" before Randy said he had to talk with the man privately. I was left with the man's girlfriend, a stranger to me. We took a seat at the tiny bar and started making small talk. "So, how long have you and Randy been together?" she asked.

Excuse me, what? I could not believe she assumed he and I were together. *Did he tell them we were together?* It was one thing to pretend to be together for the casino's sake, but if he was introducing me to friends from his past as his girlfriend, that was crossing a different line. My body froze with fear.

I said nothing in response. I knew if I told this woman Randy was my stepdad, it would embarrass him. I was at his mercy, in a foreign place, fearing for my safety. Maybe she had just assumed we were together, but I couldn't ask such a question. I was left to wrestle with the ambiguity, trying to appear older, wearing lots of makeup, sitting at a bar where I had arrived holding Randy's hand.

The two men returned and we didn't stay long. Randy didn't tell me what they did in the other room and it was the last I saw of that couple.

We proceeded to the theater where I was meant to witness greatness, to be inspired, and perhaps see a vision of my future self. I carried on with this supposed purpose of our trip, happy to step back into the fun and fantasy of it all.

We were shown to our seats at a small table close to the stage. I could feel the cheerful anticipation as the crowd started to fill. A waitress appeared wearing something like a bathing suit and an ice-skating costume rolled into one. Randy asked for a vodka cranberry and I ordered a coke.

Soon, the lights went down and the music soared. What felt like hundreds of women started pouring onto the stage. At first, I was taken with the symmetry of the choreography, like an M.C. Escher print had come to life. But as it went on, all I could see were half-naked women. I felt sad watching the make-up caked faces that erased any identity of the dancers except their height and breast size. I couldn't believe the big event Randy had brought me here for was a topless show. How could he have thought I would enjoy this, or see it as a reflection of my future self? I was neither inspired nor impressed.

I knew I had to *seem* impressed, to be grateful for the expensive tickets and excellent seats. When I even hinted at my distaste during intermission, I could feel Randy's anger. The sharpness of his voice warned me to steer clear of that side of him. Especially as we went back to our room that night.

I opened my suitcase and gathered the clothes I had packed for bed: baggy yellow sweatpants and an extra-large grey sweatshirt. I was 5'2" and 115 pounds—swimming in rolled sleeves and pant cuffs the size of inner tubes, but the fabric helped to insulate me as I left the bathroom.

Randy was reading in a chair across the room as I pulled back the covers. I exaggerated my exhaustion and laid so close to the edge of the bed, I might have fallen off. My body was positioned away from him and facing the wall as I said, "Good night," clutching the maroon bedspread tightly to my chin.

I don't remember him getting into bed but recall waking up to him lying next to me in the middle of the night. His naked back appeared like a mountain and I assumed he was only wearing underwear beneath the sheets. As far as I know, he stayed on his side of the bed the entire night and he woke up the next morning before me, dressed and ready to go. Nothing happened. He didn't touch me.

The next day was much like the first, with another show planned for the evening: Wayne Newton. But before we left that night, Randy said another old friend, Tom, was joining us for dinner.

Tom met us at our hotel room. He and Randy were chatting, then Tom waved and said, "Hi, Ingrid," from the hallway.

"Hi, Tom, it's nice to meet you," I responded from the far end of the room. Then Randy said goodbye and closed the door. "What happened?" I asked. "Isn't he coming to dinner?"

"No, I guess he had other plans and just stopped by to say hi," Randy replied.

The abrupt change seemed odd, but I was relieved I wouldn't need to navigate my ambiguous role in front of another old friend. It was becoming exhausting to be me in Vegas, and I was ready to leave as we headed for the airport the next morning.

Sitting in another taxi, my new clothes reeked from the smoke-filled air. The feeling of adventure had waned and there was largely silence between Randy and me. His mood had shifted from when we first arrived, like he was a different person. It had the effect of making me feel I had done something wrong. Like I had failed.

Based on the scenario he'd painted days before, the weekend should have been a huge success. We glimpsed "true entertainers" just as he promised.

I had gotten through "unscathed" in the sense that he didn't touch me. I know a part of me interpreted this to mean that nothing happened *at all* that weekend. Like because he didn't try to sleep with me, it really was the innocent trip I was hoping for.

But his icy demeanor, and the emptiness it created inside of me, reflected the story I had known deep down. Randy never wanted to rape me. He wanted me to want him, to fall in love with him. While I did my best to maintain his affection, it was clear I never wanted him to cross that line. It felt to me like Randy was the one who had failed that weekend, but he thought I was to blame.

Neither one of us would ever win. No matter how much I tolerated, I would never be taken care of just because. And no matter what he gave me, I would never give him all of me.

We returned to Colorado where Randy promised to tell our family what we had done, but we were home less than twenty-four hours when my mom called from Texas. She needed Randy to help drive my grandparents back to Denver, and that is what he did.

I imagined he would tell her at some point on that trip. But when they got home, I kept waiting for a sign that never came. Two months later, my grandfather died and my reality was effortlessly hidden behind Randy's role of supportive husband. He moved forward as though nothing ever happened.

A part of me started second-guessing my own sanity as the summer came and went. I kept wishing I knew someone who saw us in Vegas, to validate that the trip even happened. *What did it look like to them? What did the woman at the reception desk think? Did he really parade me around like a girlfriend?* But there was no one to ask. No one to reflect my experience.

Randy never spoke of it. My mom didn't know about it. So, I was stuck in a loop of questions, feeling dizzy as I continued living with multiple narratives of a life, and a self, that never fit together.

9

A Musician's Musician

Engaging with my family often felt like standing on the edge of a tornado, waiting to get sucked in. Even just leaving my bedroom, my body would feel the threat. But in order to have connection, or even breakfast, I had to walk directly into the storm.

I left as much of myself on solid ground as I could, through dissociation, armor, knowing it was temporary and I just had to get through it. And then the spinning would start. I'd get sucked into the center where it's almost impossible to see where "functional" and "dysfunctional" intersect. We were still going to school, our parents were going to work, everything just seemed "normal," but my body knew it wasn't.

I knew there had to be stability somewhere. I saw evidence of it outside my home. But inside, I mostly experienced the whirlwind. Why would I bring up Las Vegas with all of that going on? And when, on occasion, the wind stopped blowing, why would I stir up trouble then? So, I didn't. And neither did Randy. It was like the trip never happened.

I just kept living my life, trying to survive until I could get out of the storm for good, leaning into anything that made me feel special, hopeful, or sane. And for me, that was music.

MAD Company (Music and Dance) was Aspen High School's choir. We were a travelling rock and roll show, curating huge performances several times a year and touring on spring break to places like Disneyland.

Since my freshman year, I was one of the stars of those shows. I was mentioned in *The Aspen Times* and people always pulled me aside to say how much they enjoyed my performance. I loved that version of myself, in the eyes of people who adored me. In the eyes of people who saw me for me.

I recall hearing pure silence in our school auditorium one afternoon. I was standing by myself in the center of a bright spotlight and couldn't see my friend Roy, the sound engineer, but heard him say he was ready for me.

Roy was testing out new equipment in our newly built theatre. There was no audience, but it was the first time I was singing from such an impressive stage, and my body perceived it as the big time. Holding a cordless microphone in my hand, I was free to fill the space however I wanted.

Amazing Grace instinctively fell from my lips with notes that lingered long in the air. My voice was clearer and louder than I'd ever heard. Roy accentuated the sound, tweaking knobs on his control board, making me feel more powerful than was ever possible in the rest of my life. I felt like a gymnast, propelling myself higher and higher before sticking the perfect landing.

Nothing matched that form of expression. I could be full of self-doubt outside of that building but when I got on stage, I was a force. I commanded attention and it didn't scare me, because it was safe to take up space in the center of a song.

***

Randy's black and white headshot from 1985 was prominently placed in our home. It was framed with the announcement, "In the lounge tonight" and sitting atop a stand you might see in a hotel lobby. If he'd had a more accurate view of himself, his constant piano playing might have been tolerable, but he thought he was Elton John. He thought he was doing us a favor. It was more than the sound, it was an energetic overtaking of the house, as though nobody else lived there.

He thought of himself as a "musician's musician," implying a mastery level of technical insight and complexity. I thought he was the quintessential lounge lizard, with too much vibrato and every song sounding the same. His musical selections never changed much, so I cringe to this day when "Just Once" by James Ingram comes on the radio.

People who didn't really know me said how lucky I was, as a budding singer, to have a musician as a stepdad. One who had me singing in bars with him at age fourteen: "Such an opportunity!" But singing with Randy never really felt like it was for *me*.

I hated the way he used our shared interest to create intimate moments, like when he had me sing the duet *Somewhere Out There*. I would stand by his side, blending our voices into one.

> *Somewhere out there, if love can see us through*
> *Then we'll be together somewhere out there*
> *Out where dreams come true*

Eventually, singing with him just felt disgusting. Like he was pimping me out for his own pleasure. And yet, it was better than being ignored or punished. Better than being a reluctant audience member.

I couldn't wait to get out of there. But Randy wanted his hooks in my future too. I had started ordering college catalogs and several large envelopes from liberal arts schools with strong music programs began arriving, mostly from New York.

There were about twenty stacked on my desk when my mom came back to my room. She and I had never talked about college. I was just doing what my friends were doing, with the help of the school's college counselor.

"Ingrid, we can't afford to send you to any of those schools," she said. "You have a bit of money that your dad and I set aside for you when we divorced, but that's it."

My cheeks felt flushed and I began to shrink. I had been carrying on as though I was moving to New York for school. I took a few deep breaths, staring at my shoes while I digested what she was saying. Then I became angry we hadn't talked about it sooner. I had let myself dive into the photos of those campuses, imagining taking the train into the city. I'd built an entire new life in my mind, walking the great green lawns, and in one minute, it was gone.

"The catalogs have been coming for weeks, why are we just talking about this now?" I cried.

"I know. I'm sorry," my mom said.

Randy came to my room the next day. "Your mom told me you were pretty upset about not having money for school," he said.

I had no intention of recreating the crushing moment with him.

"Well, I have a proposition." He was trying to get eye contact, but I kept looking at the floor.

"Listen," he continued. "If you go to Berklee College of Music in Boston, I'll pay for it. Your tuition and living expenses. It's the best music school in the country for jazz and blues."

What was he saying? They suddenly had the money to send me to school?

"But if you decide to go anywhere else, you're on your own."

I began to seethe. It wasn't that they couldn't send me to school, it was that he *wouldn't*, unless I did exactly what he wanted.

I had a Berklee catalog sitting on my desk. I knew Randy's daughter Stacy had gone there (and that he didn't pay for it). And I knew immediately that I was not going to take that deal. I was not going to let him dictate my path or keep me tethered to him in this way. The conversation felt like the invitation to Vegas, only this was four more years of strings I was desperate to cut.

But I didn't say any of that. I let him think this was amazing and I was grateful. That he was a big shot, and I was so lucky... so I could enjoy a few moments of peace around the house. So he would leave my room in a good mood.

10

Ding

While my friends got the English and math awards at our assemblies, I received the music and weight training awards. I almost failed my freshman year because my goals at school were to get out of the house and be with my friends. It was so much "work" being at home, I couldn't concentrate anywhere else.

I'd earned the nickname "Ding" in Algebra class one day—short for "Dingy Ingy" and the result of asking a dumb question the whole class thought was hilarious. From that moment, to my friends, family, and teachers, it was as though my name was never actually "Ingrid." I didn't take offense. I knew it was a term of endearment. I wore it as a symbol of being accepted and loved. But I did think it was *accurate*.

I received a lot of lectures from my parents about my grades, but no one seemed to care what I was actually learning. So, I figured out how to either cheat or do the bare minimum.

The only time Randy commented on my aptitude was when he made me write an essay on "respect." I took on the task happily, and really applied myself. I turned the tables onto him, dissecting all the ways I was *disrespected* by a man who would dare have me write such an essay.

"Who wrote this?" he asked, his voice laced with suspicion.

I started burning up inside. *Who do you think wrote it? Our closest neighbor is frostbite distance. Thanks for the vote of confidence, asshole!* I knew he wasn't going to give me any credit, so I stopped trying. Even when I showed I could be brilliant, maybe especially then, I was disregarded. If I were the first female president, it wouldn't have been enough. It wouldn't prove my worth to my parents and it wouldn't give me an accurate view of myself.

So, I happily accepted myself as "Ding" and poured myself into music and my social life. I loved my group of girlfriends, although I never invited any of them over for dinner or sleepovers. I think most of them never knew where I lived. I always jumped at the chance to go to *their* houses. I felt safer almost anywhere than the place I called "home." But it was only allowed in small doses.

Another of Randy's rules—only one fun thing a week. If I stayed at a friend's house on Friday, I could not go to the movies on Saturday. To this day, I feel like I'm doing something wrong or that I'm going to get in trouble if I have fun on consecutive days.

***

Living with constant rules and stress made me want to check out from reality. So, even though I despised my parents' drinking, it was the first thing I did when I got out of the house.

Mita and I often participated in the same ritual. We would meet up with friends on a Friday or Saturday night, party at one of their houses or somewhere in the mountains, and then drive back to her house in Snowmass Village.

I would be too drunk to drive, so she would get behind the wheel and keep it in park while we lit two Marlboro Lights. We cracked the windows about an inch and then turned off the radio while Mita said an earnest prayer: "God, please bring us home safely tonight." Then, by some miracle, we made it back to her house every time.

One of the most epic nights of my high school drinking career happened shortly after the start of my senior year. My friend's parents were out of town, so with red solo cups full of beer or shots of Jägermeister, we were having a party and dreaming up our senior prank.

"Why don't we go joy riding on the golf carts at the Snowmass Club?" one of the guys said.

"What?!" We all discounted the idea. I'd never heard of anyone taking golf carts out for a spin and it seemed too rebellious. Mita was clear that she did not like this plan. Everyone in Snowmass knew her family. The Club was like their second home. "I'm out," she said.

But I was having so much fun and didn't want it to end. Several others were starting to make a plan, so seven of us drove out to Snowmass and met up in the parking lot.

"How are we going to get the carts out?" I asked when I saw they were surrounded by chains.

"We just lift them over," one of the guys said.

"Right, we just lift hundreds of pounds over the chains." My girlfriends and I started laughing as the reality began to settle in: *joy riding means stealing.*

One by one, we lifted the carts to freedom while the guys got them started with a paperclip. Soon we were headed for the rolling hills of the course. It was too dark to see and the grass was wet with dew, so we started playing accidental bumper cars until, off in the distance, we noticed a flashlight panning the course and we took off running.

Eventually, the Snowmass police took us all into the station and we had to call our parents, but there was no way I was calling mine. I couldn't imagine the wrath I'd get for something like this, so I made up a lie on the spot. "My parents are out of town, so I'm staying with my older brother, Sean," I said.

The officers didn't question my story so I called Sean, telling him what happened and, "because I'm staying with you…"

Sean took the hint, but I could tell he was pissed. "Jesus, Fea. Okay, I'll be there soon."

I was so relieved. Sean arrived and brought my friend and I, who also told the police she was staying with him, back to her house, where we stayed for the night.

By the time school started the next morning, everyone knew what had happened and no one was laughing. There were 375 students in the entire school, so news traveled fast, but I thought I'd gotten away with it as far as my parents were concerned, until we heard the Snowmass Club wanted to press charges.

This was not going to bode well.

11

The Confession

The timing of the senior prank couldn't have been worse. I had started to share some of my home life with my school counselor, Karen. She told me she was a mandated reporter of child abuse and neglect, and that what I had already shared was verging on reportable. I hadn't even told her about Vegas, and now there was a new incident with Randy that seemed much worse. I finally felt ready to tell her everything, right as I was being labelled a criminal.

Randy and I had been the only ones home one afternoon when I walked through his bedroom towards the sliding glass door, the main one we used to go in and out of the house. "Hey, can we talk for a minute?" he asked.

"Sure," I said as he motioned for me to take a seat. There was no other furniture, so I sat on the bottom edge of their waterbed. Randy sat a couple feet away, on the same side of the wooden frame, and I was creeped out before he started speaking. *What is this? Did he find out about the Snowmass Club?*

He didn't seem angry and his voice had a confessional quality. "Listen, I know there are times when I ignore you and then I seem to have a change of heart," he said.

What? I could not believe he was admitting he gave me the silent treatment.

"I see so much of myself in you," he continued. "You are so talented and I feel like we are kindred souls."

What is happening? I felt some hope and relief, that maybe he was admitting I wasn't crazy. But it was closely followed by repulsion. I loathed that he was linking us together in this cosmic way. It made me physically nauseous.

"I have so much love for you, Ingrid. I honestly wish I could give you the world."

The waterbed frame was digging into the back of my legs, pins and needles running towards my toes. I concentrated on the numbness, hoping it would spread towards my chest as Randy went on to say that his overwhelming love and longing would eventually lead to guilt and despair.

"I know these feelings are wrong," he said. "They're not the feelings one has for a stepdaughter." He then shared with me that when he felt guilty, he would have to shut me out. It was his only defense.

His clarity was astounding. I stared down at my lifeless legs, unable to move. I couldn't believe Randy knew what he was doing, and he was telling me about it so succinctly. There was so much turbulence in my chest, and I was trying to sort it out as quickly as I could.

In some ways, this was the moment I was waiting for. He was admitting that he had either been pursuing me, or hating me for it. But in other ways, I was furious he was having this conversation with me and not someone else. *What do you want me to do with this information? I just turned seventeen.*

I wished I could have said, *This has been so scary and awful,* but there was no room for my vulnerability. It's hard to explain how something could be so much about me, and not about me at all. This wasn't a confession, it felt like coercion. He wanted me to appreciate *his* vulnerability, how hard this was on him. He saw himself as a victim. It felt like Randy wanted me to take care of him, maybe tell him, *You don't have to be so hard on yourself, it's okay to love me "that way."*

I felt like the only stable person in the room when I looked up and managed to say, "I'm glad you're talking about these feelings, but I'm probably not the most appropriate person to tell." What I wanted to scream was, *Go to therapy, FUCKING ASSHOLE! This is the most inappropriate conversation I've ever had!*

Despite my attempt to offer gratitude for his candor, and to redirect his honesty, I could see he felt rejected and that it quickly turned to anger. The entire scenario he had just revealed was playing out like a movie on his face: he loved me and then he hated me. Between the two of us, I was the bad guy.

His eyes turned black and seemed to scream, *How dare you!* Then he got up to leave. Surprisingly, I didn't want him to go. I detested Randy, but returning to the angry silent treatment was so much worse. And despite the dysfunction, I still had a longing to be taken care of and loved like a normal girl in a normal family. It seemed like such a simple request. *Why can't you just love me like a stepdaughter?*

"Randy, wait!" I said. "What did you expect me to do with all of that?" Maybe if he remembered how young I was, he wouldn't be so mad. Maybe he would remember that he wanted to give me the world and it wouldn't have to be so conditional.

He kept walking away, out of the room, and I was left sitting on his bed. Too stunned to cry, or even move, I stared off into space. A couple minutes later, I heard him playing piano and it brought me back to the pins and needles poking my skin.

This is not okay. I can't keep living like this.

***

I had come to trust my counselor, Karen. She had a way of eliciting what was *really* going on. I went to her cubicle shortly after Randy's confession. Quiet in my approach, as I didn't want to disturb her, I peeked around the fabric partition to get her attention.

Karen invited me in and I swallowed hard to give myself a moment of composure before finally telling her everything: How Randy had taken me to Vegas eight months earlier, how it felt like he wanted me to be his girlfriend and he never told my mom about the trip. I told her about Randy's awareness of his feelings and how he knew he ignored me for months when he felt guilty. I had already told her about my parents' drinking and how it scared my brothers and me. And after I said all of this, Karen said, "Ingrid, this is reportable. I need to call social services."

The gravity of her reaction was a relief. It felt like my first taste of sanity in a very long time. *This is reportable.*

"Rather than talking to a social worker on my own, I'd like for you to be there," she said. Karen thought it might give me a sense of "agency" if I personally reported everything that had been happening. "I have to make a report no matter what, but why don't you take a little time to think about how you'd like to do it."

Karen also suggested we could invite my mom to the meeting, so she could have a chance to process it before we brought Randy in. That sounded like a good idea. It felt like Karen was thinking about things from my mom's point of view, trying to give her some agency, too.

"I think that sounds fine, let me just think about it for the rest of the day," I said before leaving Karen's cubicle. I walked down the hall towards my locker and saw the payphone at the edge of the hallway. I often called my dad from that phone, because I had more privacy in public than I did at home.

I decided I should tell him what was going on. My dad still lived in Denver with his wife, Alice. When I called him during the day, I could catch him on his 1-800 number at work, where I felt like he had more privacy too.

I never got along with Alice. It seemed like she had a grudge against me from the beginning. Like she resented me for not rolling out the welcome mat. But we each had to tolerate one another if we wanted to be in relationship with my dad.

My dad was still a drinker, and he met Alice in a bar shortly after my mom moved in with Randy. She wasn't just a mean drunk, she could be vicious. One time, I was sitting in their living room, watching TV when she came in, slurring, "I know you slept with Randy."

This came out of nowhere. I'd never even spoken with her about Randy. *What is she talking about?!*

Given the facts of my homelife in Aspen, her comment was painful enough, but it was the way she implied *I* was sleeping with *him* … like I had seduced my stepdad. In truth, I was a virgin. I had never seduced anyone. I started crying as I told Alice this, but she never heard me and she never apologized. She continued to see me through a painfully critical lens, and tried to convince my dad on many occasions of what she thought she saw.

Whenever I talked to my dad about how Alice treated me, he would always apologize on her behalf. He would tell me she'd been abused in her previous marriages. I hated that he defended her, but at least he didn't make me feel like a liar.

I picked up the payphone receiver at school and stared at the silver coil. After a few rings, I heard my dad's voice. "Hey kiddo!"

I immediately started to cry and couldn't hide it. "Hi, Dad," I sobbed.

"What's going on, Ingrid?"

He already knew I didn't like Randy. Neither did he. The betrayal of losing his wife to his best friend had to cut deep. But my dad didn't know about Vegas, so I told him everything, just like I'd told Karen.

"Do you want me to come and get you?" he asked. I knew he meant it and if I wanted him to get in his car and drive four hours to pick me up, he would have. But I didn't want that. I didn't want to move to Denver. I didn't have any community or friends, I wouldn't have had the musical opportunities that held me together. I wanted to finish my senior year in Aspen and I wanted Randy to get in trouble for what he had done.

"You don't have to come," I said. "I just needed you to know what was going on. I'm going to call social services with my counselor and they'll help us sort everything out." I was comforted knowing my dad was there and that he loved me. "I'll let you know what happens. I'm really nervous, but I think it's the right thing to do."

"I'm here if you need anything, and I'm so sorry you are going through this," my dad said. We both said "I love you," and then I hung up.

I went to class, thinking only about what I wanted to say to my mom. The more I thought about it, the more optimistic I felt. Karen knew I didn't have bruises, but she said she *had* to make a report. She knew Randy hadn't tried to sleep with me, but it was *still* reportable. She wasn't just advocating for me, she was advocating for my mom, and it made me feel like my mom and I could finally be on the same team. I went from having a secret fantasy that Karen could be my mom, to feeling like I might be able to get my own mom back.

I went to Karen's office before I left school that day. "I'm ready to call," I said. "Can we do it tomorrow morning?"

"I'll make the arrangements," Karen said. "I'm proud of you."

12

The Intervention

When Karen arrived at school the next day, I met her in her office. "Are you ready?" she asked.

"No," I said honestly as she gave me a nod of understanding.

"I've already spoken with a social worker and she's available to come to school whenever I tell her we're ready."

"Okay, I guess we should do this. But now there's something else I need to tell you." It had been made clear to me that the Snowmass Club expected us to work off the damages to their property on the weekends. I was going to have to tell my parents what happened.

Karen seemed as sad about the reality as I was, but we agreed I should just lay everything out once my mom came to school. "Okay, deep breaths," I said. "Let me call my mom."

I forced my arm out of paralysis to reach for Karen's phone. Before we called the social worker, I needed to ask my mom if she could come to the school. She was at the office with Randy, so I was terrified he might answer the phone or be standing a few feet away.

Don't forget to breathe.

I heard my mom pick up and was so relieved. "Hi, Mom, it's me. I'm wondering if it would be possible for you to come to the school right now and not tell Randy where you are going?"

"Why, what's going on?" she said. "Is everything okay?"

I told her everything was fine but I needed to talk to her by herself.

She was hesitant. "I don't understand."

"I know, but you will when you get here. Can you just please come? I need you to come by yourself and not say anything to Randy." I was either closing my eyes tightly or lost all focus. Everything seemed black.

"Okay, just give me a few minutes," she said.

I couldn't read her tone. Was she mad, or trying to sound neutral so she didn't give anything away? My stomach was in knots. I hung up the phone. "She's coming," I told Karen. "But I think she's mad I put her in that position." The last thing I wanted was for my mom to be angry. I was already second guessing this plan.

Twenty minutes later, I saw my mom pull up around the same time as two women from social services. Karen and I met everyone in the front office. My mom looked so nervous, I wanted to reach out and tell her everything would be okay, but I said nothing except "Hello" while Karen and the school secretary led us to a private room that looked like a long, deep closet with chairs stacked inside. I could feel my heartbeat at least three feet in front of my chest.

We all grabbed a chair and took a seat in a circle. I suddenly felt claustrophobic as I scanned the room for any sign of support. All eyes were on me, and then Karen made quick introductions before giving me the floor.

"Thanks for coming, Mom. I know this is weird and there is a lot I want to share, but first ..."

I had to tell her about the Snowmass Club. It felt like an easier thing to start with and I just wanted to get it out of the way. I finished with the part about having to do community service and could tell my mom was pissed. She didn't say she was angry, but she didn't have to. I could feel *her* heart beating three feet in front of her chest, like it was reaching out to pummel me.

"But that's not really why we are here," I continued. I had to take the plunge. "It's all terrible timing, but..."

I looked over at Karen, trying to reconnect with a "normal" reaction to my homelife.

"When you left for Texas to be with Grandma and Grandpa, Randy surprised me with a trip to Las Vegas. He wouldn't let me tell anyone about it, including you, and he made me lie to the boys about where we were going."

Once I started talking, I couldn't stop.

"He bought me lots of clothes and gifts and made me hold his hand everywhere we went. We only had one hotel room, with a huge king-sized bed. It felt like a suite and there was a mirror on the ceiling. Randy said he would tell you about the trip, but I don't think he ever did. Did he?" The question surprised me. I didn't intend to ask it.

My mom's body seemed affixed to her chair. She barely moved a muscle but was able to shake her head "No" about an inch side to side.

"I didn't think so," I replied. "Then, Randy recently had a talk with me when you weren't home. He admitted he was in love with me, and when he feels guilty about it, he shuts me out with the silent treatment. There are times when he doesn't look at me or speak one word to me for months. I'm sure you've seen that happen."

I felt like a plug had been pulled from my storehouse of secrets and the water just kept pouring and pouring till there was almost none left. I didn't show any emotion other than the fear that was holding me upright. No one else uttered a word as I recounted all these details and when I finally came to a stopping point, one of the social workers finally chimed in.

"Thank you for sharing all of that, Ingrid. Lynn, do you have any questions or anything you'd like to say?"

Everyone looked at my mom. There was just silence and her pursed lips. For the second time, she shook her head, "No."

The social worker continued, "Well, I understand there are two more siblings and some things we might want to discuss together, perhaps we should bring them into the room now?" She looked at Karen. I wasn't expecting this, and neither were my brothers.

Karen said, "Okay, I believe one of them is here in the high school, and the other is at the middle school, right?"

I waited to see if my mom would answer, but she didn't. "Yes, John is here and Josh is at the middle school," I replied.

"Okay, let me go to the office and I'll be right back." Karen left for the door and the social workers, my mom and I sat in awkward silence. I glanced at my mom, but she was looking down. Her body language seemed to read, *I am a stone, don't even look at me.*

My brothers were pulled out of class. Josh was walked up to the high school and then both boys came into the room with Karen. We grabbed two more chairs and one of the social workers told them why we were all there and asked me if they knew about the trip to Vegas.

"No," I replied.

It seemed like another pause inviting me to share, so I told the boys what had happened. John seemed like he knew something was up that weekend, but he didn't offer any more details in the meeting. The social worker asked my brothers how they felt in our home and if there was anything they wanted to say.

"Well, I don't like Randy's temper," Josh said. Then he shared a recent story of hearing him hit our mom, screaming at her in their bedroom. Josh ran in to see what was going on and found our mom crouched in the corner, crying and begging Randy to stop.

I remembered driving home that night and seeing several cop cars driving away from the direction of our house. I thought, *I hope they weren't just there*. It was dark and quiet when I walked in our front door, and then I heard Josh whispering from the loft up above, "Ing, Ing," trying to get my attention.

I climbed up the ladder and he told me he had grabbed a baseball bat from the living room and went into our parents' room swinging and yelling, "Get the hell away from her!" before calling 911. Josh was fourteen and growing into his broad shoulders and chiseled jaw. I worried that one day the bat might swing back at him.

Josh told the social workers that the police came and went with no report. Our mom didn't want to press charges. So, everyone had gone to bed and the next morning, acted like nothing had happened. Josh looked over at our mom with the tenderness of a little boy and an expression that seemed to say, *Sorry, Mom*.

John admitted that he hated our parents' drinking. He said we were all afraid to be in the car with them and always nervous what might happen next.

Then there was a long pause.

I did it, I thought. I told her everything and I'm finally going to hear my mom say, "I'm so sorry, sweetie. I had no idea. That must have been so scary." Maybe she'd give me a hug, pulling me close to protect me from any more hurt. Maybe she'd be angry with Randy, so angry she couldn't contain herself, screaming, "How could he do this to me and my family?! How could I have been so forgiving and blind?!"

But my mom didn't do or say any of those things. Through her pursed lips, and tears she was struggling to hold back, her only response was, "I don't want to talk about this anymore without my husband. Randy needs to be here right now."

In that moment, I knew our intervention had failed. Nothing was going to cut through the fog my mom was living in. Nothing was going to give her a sense of agency. It was like she wasn't even there, like I had no mother at all.

13

The Talking Stick

The social workers suggested we all take a break and that my mom call Randy to come to the school. Josh, John and I went outside while we were waiting. I could hardly walk, I was so stunned. My brothers both seemed nervous that Randy was on his way, and I guess I was too, it just felt like I was dead inside.

Since our parents' business wasn't far, we went back to the small office and waited with all the grownups. They were trying to have regular conversation and I understood the impulse, but it felt really insensitive. I did not want to engage in small talk.

I sat directly across from my mom again and she wouldn't look at me. There wasn't an ounce of softening. Then Randy was shown into our room. He stood in the doorway and I could tell he was furious. Once he saw there was an empty seat next to my mom, he stomped in and sat down. "What's going on here?" he snarled.

Karen gave some orientation and thankfully shared many of the details from our initial meeting. I don't think I could have said them all again. Randy was huffing and hissing at each remark, and with every utterance, I shrank. Eventually, one of the social workers asked if he would like to explain his side of the story.

"Can I talk now?" His sharp tone implied the absurdity of being asked to sit through such a diatribe. "I can't believe you had this little meeting without me, but it's my turn to talk now." He pointed directly at me as he gave a hard stare to the social workers and Karen. "Ingrid is a spoiled brat. She's just upset that we give her chores and make her take out the trash. She's angry that we don't give her as much freedom as she thinks her friends have. This is all bullshit. I know that the kids don't love the time we spend at The Tavern, but nothing else is true."

Randy went into denial and a full-scale character assassination of me while squeezing my mom's hand. I saw she was squeezing his back, staring directly at him.

Every fiber of my body started to collapse. I was getting smaller and smaller, darker and deeper, until there was nothing left. Randy made me question my own sanity and the smear campaign he unleashed amplified the results. This all felt so much worse than keeping it quiet and to myself. I wanted them to see my pain, but instead I was seen as a liar, as insignificant. I wanted to evaporate.

"I know this was difficult," one of the social workers said after Randy finished, and I could have laughed at the understatement, but I was too numb. She thanked us all for sharing our experience and then said they needed some time to make a recommendation before we all stood to leave the closet-like room.

Randy said goodbye to John before marching off towards the parking lot. My mom exchanged a few words with Josh—it seemed like reassurance was being offered between them—then followed Randy. No one said anything to me as I watched them all leave and then walked with Karen in silence back to her office.

"That was brutal," I said as I slumped in a chair. There were no tears, no big reactions, I just felt like a huge ice cream scoop had scraped out my insides. Karen didn't seem to have words either, but her face told me she understood.

***

As usual, everyone in my family kept on like nothing happened until we got the call from social services. My mom gave me the news in passing, standing in the kitchen, that we had to go to family therapy. I could tell she was angry about it, angry with me.

"We all have to go?" I asked.

"Yes, we're mandated to family therapy," she huffed.

It felt pathetic. I felt pathetic. No one was being removed from the home, no one was asking for a divorce, or going to jail. We just needed a supportive environment to come together as a family. *Yeah, right.*

In a small town like Aspen, there weren't many choices for therapists. So, if you needed one, chances are you saw Cindy, who worked out of her home, nestled on the side of Brush Creek Mountain.

On Saturday, all five of us piled in the minivan and drove to our first session in silence. When we arrived, Cindy showed us to her living room-style office, populated with large furniture arranged in a circle. The dark walls reflected the mood of my family as we filed in. Cindy's cheery and optimistic disposition made her seem out of place and made me wonder if she was up to the task.

Wearing a fitted, Scandinavian wool sweater and sensible shoes, Cindy stood to the side of the brown, leather chair where Randy was sitting. It felt like the two of them were at the head of the table, even though there wasn't one.

After some quick introductions, Cindy asked us to share with her what brought us to her office. She understood some details from the social workers, but wanted to hear our perspective.

Randy began by looking directly at me. "Ingrid, I can't believe because of you and your lies, we are all here today." He was furious.

It's hard to imagine I was surprised by this, and yet I felt stunned that he chose to maintain the lie. It horrified me and made me spring into action. *Maybe if I can convince Cindy, she will make my mom see.*

I launched in with more details about Vegas, about the women who threw their panties on stage at Wayne Newton, and how dirty our fingers were from playing the slot machines. *How would I know any of these things if I'd never been to Vegas!*

Randy said matter-of-factly, "That's all a figment of your imagination."

At this point, John chimed in. "I know you didn't go out of town on business, Dad." He said he remembered seeing Randy pick me up from school that day. He saw us walking to the car and tried to run after us, but got there too late.

It felt like John had joined me in this tug-o-war, bringing the rope back to center. Despite his loyalty to his dad, John was on my side. At least he seemed to believe me.

But Randy made up a new lie on the spot, "I was coming to find you that day, son."

What? This made no sense. Find John for what? To take him to Vegas? When he was going on a business trip?

John pushed back, and Randy seemed to get more enraged, like he was being backed into a corner. Randy started talking in circles that made no sense, but one thing became clear: losing John's allegiance just about made him burst. I think Cindy saw it, too, because she rested her hand on Randy's shoulder, maybe trying to calm him a bit.

Watching her calmed *me* a bit. She was still the only person standing in the room and it gave her an air of authority. I hoped Randy would take her cue to bring down his tone.

In fact, her touch infuriated him and he yelled, "Don't put your hands on me!"

Cindy visibly jumped back, the color draining from her face. She took a breath and calmly apologized. "Let's all take a moment," she said. Then she indicated that she wanted to give everyone in the room a chance to speak and invoked the idea of a "talking stick." Perhaps if one person at a time was given the floor, we could really listen to one another. I suspected as a way to give Randy some power that he felt slipping away, she started with him. "Why don't you go around the room and tell each person what you'd like to say in this environment, and then everyone else will take a turn after you?"

Randy began by turning his attention back to John. "John, you've always been my favorite child," he said.

Randy had two other biological children and was sitting in a room with two of his stepchildren. *This is what he chose to say?* I was disgusted and looked over at Josh, who had a blank stare on his face.

Then Randy turned to Josh and said nothing of consequence. It felt like John was the angel, Josh was invisible, and I was the scapegoat for everything.

When Randy turned to me, he said, "Ingrid, I wish you would stop all of this. You're being so selfish with these lies and I can't understand what you're hoping to gain."

My chest was swelling with fury, but I swallowed hard, waiting for my turn with the imaginary stick.

Cindy invited my mom to share next. She turned to Josh first. "Josh, you've always been my favorite child."

Is this how family therapy is supposed to go? I looked at Cindy to see if she was going to say something, to come to my rescue, but she didn't. I wanted to cry out, but I didn't feel safe enough to feel those feelings, so I just let the tears roll up behind my eyes.

I was still reeling when my mom turned to me. "Ingrid, I believe that you believe those things happened with Randy, but I don't believe they did."

That sentence: *I believe that you believe those things happened with Randy, but I don't believe they did.*

She didn't want to call me a liar, so she made me delusional instead.

"Mom, why would I make this all up?!" I yelled. "I wouldn't have *anything* to gain by making up such a story!"

It fell on deaf ears. We started to argue again and Cindy tried to bring down the levels in the room but offered no meaningful interventions. We simply destroyed one another with a talking stick. Josh made the most coherent point of the day when he said, "Why should I say anything? I'll just get home and be in worse trouble and no one will be there to deal with it but me."

He was right. The game of pin the blame made things worse. The five of us got back into our minivan and drove home in silence.

As soon as it felt safe to leave my room, I went to John's and thanked him for trying to stand up for me. He told me he was certain his dad and my mom would divorce. "What parent can stand by knowing their husband made sexual advances towards their daughter?"

I wished his premonition were true, that my mom eventually saw things the way he did. But the only thing derived from therapy was that I was a liar, that asking for help makes things worse, that I had a predator for a stepdad—and a mother who didn't believe me.

It was like I'd been on a roller coaster, slowly ticking up, up, up for the past several years. The hot tub when I was 13. My parents drinking. The silent treatment and constantly being grounded. Vegas. Higher and higher the coaster climbed until I called social services. That moment was like being parked at the highest point of the ride. We could all see the entire landscape around us. I was certain everyone would see the same things, the danger and the terror.

My entire being was ready to fall over the crest of the hill, ready to scream and let it all go, knowing it was about to come to an end. I'd finally arrive at a place of rest, a place of safety and calm. I could get off the ride.

But the coaster never came down. At least not for me. All that anxiety was bottled up with no release, like I was stuck on "high." I couldn't relax or switch off without alcohol or drugs. I was hypervigilant, on edge and waiting for the next terrible thing to happen. All the while doubting myself. Doubting what my own body knew, perched dangerously high above the ground. Telling myself their version of the story, one that fit the unthinkable outcome I was living.

I didn't have bruises.
She never left him.
He didn't actually rape me.
Maybe I wasn't worth believing.
Maybe it wasn't that bad.

14

Tell Them You're an Orphan

Not long after therapy, both Josh and John decided to move out. John went to live with his mom in Carbondale, staying in the Aspen School district, and Josh went to Denver to live with our dad. I only had a few months left of high school and couldn't imagine leaving before graduation. I slipped into a kind of autopilot, no longer deluding myself that things could change. Just willing myself to survive it all a little longer.

Randy and I didn't have many interactions after my brothers moved out, but he continued his seesaw behavior: mostly despising me, then crossing more boundaries.

There were times he stood outside my bathroom when I showered. As the water fell on my long, brown hair, I'd hear a ferocious knock on the door. "I don't want you wasting so much water!" he'd yell. Then he would stand there, feet away from my naked body, counting each minute that passed. He threatened to come in and turn off the water if I didn't get out within five. I raced through my shower; furious he would invade my privacy in a way that allowed him to maintain his "innocence" once again.

One morning I went out to my car and saw I had a flat tire. My grandparents had given me their Dodge Colt after my grandpa got sick. It was winter and the snow was softly falling, creating a little slope from the rim of my tire to the ground. I came back inside to tell my parents.

"There is a spare tire and jack in the back of your car," Randy said.

"Okay, but I don't know how to use them. I've never changed a tire and it's snowing."

"What would you do if you were stranded on the side of the road?" he asked.

I thought this might be an opportunity for someone to *teach* me such a handy skill, but in Randy's book, learning the hard way was the only sufficient method. I went back outside where I gathered the spare from my trunk and got to work, my fingers bright red and pulsing in the cold.

I could see Randy standing at the sliding glass door, watching me from the warmth of the house. When I managed to get the spare attached to the car, he instructed me to drive down to the Conoco station at the bottom of the hill—three-and-a-half miles of dirt roads and icy pavement. The attendant took one look at my car from across the lot and told me my spare was on backwards. He said he was glad I made it down the hill and couldn't believe an adult had "supervised" such a lesson.

I was truly confused in these situations. *Was this how you taught independence? Did Randy not know how to change a tire, so he avoided looking bad at any cost, even the cost to my safety?* I was constantly trying to figure out abnormal behavior through a normal lens and could never make any sense of it.

About a month later, Randy came back to my room one night. "Hey, can I come in?" He said and I met him at the door. There was something strange about him. His eyes were dark and vacant. Like his body was there, but he wasn't actually in it.

"Yeah?" I said.

Before I knew what was happening, Randy leaned in and kissed me hard on the mouth. He had never kissed me. My brain wanted to put it in a fatherly context, but it was too forceful and lasted too long. Then he pulled back to look at me. I was so shocked I didn't say anything. I smelled the alcohol on his breath and stood completely still. Then he leaned in to kiss me again.

My body sprang into action as I pushed his chest away. "Randy, stop!"

He stepped back and looked at me as though he was coming out of some possession and said, "I'm sorry." But the words had no weight to them. I felt like I was standing in front of a person who wasn't a person at all. It was terrifying.

Randy turned and walked away without saying another word. I watched him move, without urgency or purpose, and I just stood there, frozen in my doorway.

I was close to graduation, but it also felt like an eternity before I could leave. I asked my mom if I could live with Mita for the last few months of school without telling her about the kiss. She gave me a look that could have burned a hole in my face before storming off to her bedroom. When she quickly returned, she started waving my fake IDs three inches from my face.

"You aren't such a good girl! You need to take more responsibility for your own misery around here," she said as I tracked the IDs like a hawk, hoping she would set them down in a place I could stealthily steal them back. They had gone missing months earlier, only days after I received them.

"How often does Randy go through my things?" I yelled.

I was so angry she found another way to make everything my fault. It's amazing I wasn't getting in worse trouble, given my screwed-up home life, but she only saw how "bad" I was. I was nominated for prom queen, the star of our musical, I was celebrated by so many other people, but never by her. I actually thought they might be relieved to get rid of me. But I never got those IDs and they didn't let me move in with Mita.

Overwhelmed by all of it, one night I grabbed a metal nail file from my bathroom as though sleepwalking. I brought it into my bedroom and sat on the floor, between my bed and the wall. I was tucked back as far as possible from where my parents were in the house when I started to slowly saw back-and-forth on my wrist. Dust from the nail file was mixing with my burning skin and although it was starting to hurt, I kept up with the pressure and repetitive motion.

Maybe part of me wanted to see the pain I was feeling, so it would have a witness. I know I didn't want to kill myself, and that if I did, a metal nail file wouldn't do it. Maybe it was a classic cry for help, except I didn't want my parents to know what was happening. I don't think they ever did.

Mita called as I was well into this process. I heard Randy yell that she was on the phone. "I got it," I shouted quickly so he wouldn't come back to my room.

When I knew Randy had hung up, I tried having a normal conversation, but Mita knew something was off. Feeling the sting of the red and weeping wounds on both of my wrists, I started to cry. I promised Mita I would stop if she promised not to tell. But she couldn't keep the secret from her mom later that night.

The next day, I was sitting in class when I saw Mita's mom, Lollie, appear through the tiny window of my classroom door. She was looking directly at me, motioning for me to meet her in the hallway.

My sweater sleeves were tucked into my hands, hiding the bandages. I could hardly look Lollie in the eyes, I was so broken. "This has gone too far," she said.

Lollie took me to see a different therapist in town, not telling my parents. I saw that person once or twice, but didn't feel like it was helping. Everyone in "authority" seemed as powerless as me.

I somehow made it to the end of my senior year, and had been accepted to Colorado State University on a probationary status. I decided to attend with what little money had been set aside. It would get me through my freshman year if I also got a part-time job.

I was packing up my bathroom as Randy came to the door for the last conversation we had prior to my leaving. I was sitting on the tile floor, packing toiletries from under the cabinet. I actually imagined he might be coming to offer some words of wisdom. Maybe end things on a decent note. Me and my perpetual optimism.

"You should tell the kids in college you're an orphan," he said, his body rigid and menacing, "because that would be closer to the truth than the lies you've been spreading around here."

"Thanks for the pep talk," I said with all the sarcasm and contempt I could muster. Randy walked away and I quickly gathered the rest of my things, putting them in my car.

My mom came outside to see me off, teary about her daughter leaving the nest and wanting to make sure

I hadn't forgotten anything. "Did you say goodbye to Randy?" she asked.

"Yeah, Mom. We said goodbye."

I gave her a hug and got in the car. I still hadn't come down from that roller coaster, but I felt the hopefulness of driving further and further away from the source of my pain, thinking just maybe, I could leave it in those mountains.

Part Two: Trauma Responses

"The attempt to escape from pain, is what creates more pain."

— Gabor Maté

15

New Beginnings, Old Habits

Arriving at Colorado State, I didn't just want a fresh start on the outside, I wanted one on the *inside*. I tried to be "good"—I loved my new friends, sharing our dreams in freshly decorated dorms. But I didn't want to get out of bed most mornings. I didn't love my classes and when nobody knew I was missing, it was hard to go. I was in a new environment, but I brought me with me.

I had been in Fort Collins about two months when I started going to a Christian church with my new friend, Meg. There was a large band and I loved watching the other young people on Sundays. I was sitting along the back wall of the giant sanctuary one morning when a stream of tears began falling from my cheeks. "If you want to turn your will and life over to the care of God, please come down to the stage," was the repeated invitation over soft but dramatic music.

One by one, parishioners got up from their seats and proceeded to the front of the church to receive a blessing. I wanted to go with them. But I couldn't propel myself out of my seat as though I were inherently worthy. I knew that was the point—that we are all worthy—but even God couldn't save me from my shame.

No matter how much I looked like I belonged on the outside, nothing could hide the stark contrast of my insides. *I was evil.* That's how I felt about myself. And that's the feeling that held me to the back of the church and eventually stopped me from going altogether.

I quickly gained more than the "freshman fifteen" as I gorged myself on huge bowls of Lucky Charms for breakfast, lunch and dinner. I tried bingeing and purging, laxatives and diets, anything to manage my internal world via the number on the scale, but I could never get enough out. Trying to was harder than holding it all in, absorbing each calorie like a shield. The comfort that food provided seemed far more important than how I thought I was meant to avoid, control or get rid of it.

The first night I went to a party, I never made it back to the dorms. I don't recall where I slept because I was too drunk. My drinking and drug use was escalating now that every day could be "fun" if I wanted.

I quickly lost my virginity to a senior I had met on the dance floor of a party. He was goofy and handsome, and I was instantly obsessed. We slept together on our second date, and in the morning, when his roommate walked in and said, "Hey, who is that?" Christopher looked as though he wasn't sure how to answer. "It's Ingrid," he finally said. Both the roommate and I clocked his difficulty and I was devastated. Not as much by Christopher's indifference as by his roommate's smirk. She looked directly at me and laughed before walking away.

I memorized Christopher's full, middle and last name after that night, as though being able to recite it would inject some meaning into my first time. I only saw him once more after that night.

My mom and Randy never came to visit. I actually hadn't heard Randy's voice in months and didn't realize what a relief it had been until he answered the phone one day.

I was standing in my dorm with the telephone in my hand. I was sure he had been avoiding me through caller ID, but this time he picked up. "Hey, kid," he said.

I immediately began to cry and closed my eyes as if they could shut out the world. I felt as though I had just been steamrolled by Randy's voice and he was standing in my dorm, staring at my flattened remains. I couldn't believe, "Hey, kid" did that to me.

From then on, I was wary of calling home. It was like roulette. If I called too late in the day, they could be drinking and those conversations were painful but considerably easier than when *he* answered. Every time I called, I wondered: *Will they love me now, will they choose me now? Am I good enough, now?*

It never occurred to me to disconnect from them altogether. It felt like my mom's love and acceptance, and even Randy's, was the key to my happiness—the key to not being evil. I couldn't tolerate that my own mom saw me so poorly and the only way out was to convince her otherwise. To hope she would eventually see the truth. So, I kept waiting. I kept trying.

I stayed at Colorado State for one year and somehow passed my classes, but I ran out of money and didn't want to take out loans. I moved to Denver and worked at Musicland, popping cassettes out of those plastic cages for customers before becoming an administrative assistant downtown. I drank in dive bars with people twice my age, where nobody checked my fake ID. I was just existing until a hopeful thought occurred: *Maybe I can leave Colorado. Maybe I should move to New York?*

Almost anyone who had ever heard me sing suggested I try out for *Star Search*. I never wanted to be on that show, but I still wanted to be a star. I was nineteen and felt empowered by the idea I could make my own way in New York.

I made a trip to the city, just to make sure I really wanted to go through with it. Sitting in my terminal at the airport, I met a woman named Camila who was reading *The Celestine Prophecy*. We ended up chatting about synchronicities steering us down a spiritual path and later asked to sit next to one another on the plane.

We landed in the city much later than expected, so Camila wouldn't let me take the bus and subway to a friend of a friend's apartment like I'd planned. She called us a taxi and we went to her friend Manny's house in the Bronx. I was going to a stranger's house either way, as I had barely spoken to my friend's friend. At least Camila and I had spent the day together.

The cab driver's New York accent was magic and the skyline was a million times bigger and brighter than anything I had seen in the movies. It awakened a part of me I had never experienced, like I wanted to devour my surroundings, eat them, and keep them inside of me forever. I felt like I was home.

Manny was around sixty with white hair and an unsteady gait. He had a huge apartment with a spare bedroom at the end of a long hallway. He had lived there for decades, high above the Hudson River. He said I could stay with him if I decided to move, and I quickly took him up on the offer, silently musing over all the "advice" I'd received from people in Colorado before my trip. "Don't look anybody in the eye when you're walking down the street!" And yet, here I was, being completely taken care of by the first New Yorkers I had met.

16

Second Verse, Same as the First

It was Manny who came to pick me up from my second flight into the city, the day I was moving in with him. We stuffed all of my bags in his trunk and backseat before heading back to his apartment in the Bronx.

He and I fell into a routine quickly. He made me a toasted bialy in the mornings, a traditional Jewish pastry, and put it in a brown bag with a scribbled smile. I would eat my breakfast on the bus towards Manhattan. Later, as I rode the subway between employment agencies and apartments I couldn't afford, I played a little game with myself. *What if I were wearing those shoes?* Gazing down at feet from all over the world, I populated my mind with different selves I might become.

The first full-time job I landed was at a law firm in the World Trade Center. I couldn't believe my new life. Security badges gave me access to the highest floors of the towers and enough money to buy new suits in the shops on the first floor. Manny eventually helped me find my own apartment not far from his in the Bronx and I moved into the two-bedroom with a new friend, Desiree, who I happened to meet in Denver shortly before my move. She was a friend of my cousin's, and when she said she was living in New York, I scribbled her number on my arm with eyeliner and called her before my first visit.

I scoured the *Village Voice* for musical opportunities, sending headshots and demo tapes to prospective bands in the mail. My plan was to audition on nights and weekends while I worked for Richard, the Managing Partner of the firm, during the day.

Early on, I had lunch at a bustling deli across the street. I put my purse under my chair by my feet, but when I went to leave, it was gone. Strangers who saw me looking for it suggested I search the trashcans nearby in case the thief took my wallet and dumped the bag. I didn't find any trace of my belongings, my hand written address book, new sunglasses, or the badge that gave me access to the Trade Center elevators.

The building security tried calling Richard, but he wasn't there. Next they tried Stew, the office manager who also worked for Richard and was technically my boss as well. I was embarrassed they had to call him, but Stew just laughed as he told the guard I was legitimate and began leading me through the process of getting another ID.

Stew took me under his wing, like a mentor. He was in his late thirties and had lived in New York all his life. He said he loved my bravery, moving to a new place and pursuing my passion. He started inviting me to lunch and we often went to Pugsley's Pub near Wall Street.

Pugsley's was a tiny bar tucked into the corner of a high-rise hotel, just a short walk from the Trade Center. It was always full of peanut shells, male stockbrokers, and two blonde bartenders who never asked to see my ID. Stew and I found ourselves there almost daily, and eventually stopped ordering food as a pretense for the liquid lunches we were ingesting.

These daytime invitations by Stew were eventually extended to lavish parties at night. My small-town roots would show as I gawked at the elaborate décor, fancy food, music, and dancing taking place on a random Tuesday. At the end of one party, Stew was hailing me a taxi when he suddenly and forcibly stuck his tongue down my throat. I was horrified and immediately pushed him away. "Don't ever do that again!" I said. I knew he was married with kids. I saw him as a father figure.

Stew apologized and neither of us spoke about the incident the next day when we went for lunch as usual. The next Monday I arrived at work to find I had several messages from the weekend. Sitting just outside of Stew's office, the red light blinking on my phone, I glanced over at him through the glass wall and saw him leaning back in his chair, his back to me, staring out at the skyline.

I pushed play and heard Stew's voice. "I wish I was with you right now. I'm thinking about all the things I'd like to do to you..." He went on and on in a whisper, then called back ten minutes later, no doubt making sure his wife couldn't hear. He left several fantasies over voicemail and I was horrified.

I knew I could be flirtatious and I enjoyed his attention *to a point,* but I never wanted it to go this far. I thought I had made it clear I wasn't interested in him. So, when he didn't stop with the messages, I told Richard what had been happening.

He seemed appalled by Stew's actions. "If I ever saw you at a party, even as a coincidence, I would consider it inappropriate and immediately leave," Richard said as we sat in his corner office. *This is the proper boss/employee relationship,* I thought. Richard said I wouldn't have to work for Stew anymore and I was so relieved. He said it would be sorted out by the following week.

But weeks went by and I was still answering Stew's phone. When I asked Richard about it again, he admitted it was complicated and that I would have to stay at that desk, in the same role. It reinforced an old lesson I had wanted to forget: reaching out for help is a waste of time. So, I quit my steady, well-paying job and started working temp jobs all over the city.

Around the corner from Pugsley's Pub was another bar I'd often go to with friends after work. Robbie the bartender had a strong Irish brogue. He never let my glass get half empty and he never charged me for the extra pours.

I knew Robbie was engaged and I wasn't attracted to him, but I wanted to maintain his attraction and generosity. Between our constant flirtation and my intoxication, the delicate balance became hard to strike. I was very drunk as Robbie was closing up the bar one night. "You can hang out and finish your drink while I close everything up," he said as he locked the front doors.

Next thing I knew, we were in the coat closet with our pants around our ankles. It was the quickest sex of my life, and he promptly excused himself to grab paper towels from behind the bar. I watched as he got them wet and began to wash my scent off his body. I thought: *I can never come back here again.*

I knew Stew and Robbie were attracted to me. I knew that by flirting, I was playing with fire. But I naïvely imagined neither of them would ever cross the line. I perceived my job, our age difference, and the fact I would never have an affair as safe and clear boundaries. I thought Stew's marriage and Robbie's engagement kept me safe. But these men were the first of many who had no problems ignoring those lines, making me regret my ability to play so loosely with them.

Over and over again, older professors, bosses, colleagues, even Manny ... would all start out as kind, encouraging and helpful, only to eventually try and sleep with me. It happened so often, I felt like I was wearing a sign advertising my poor boundaries and need for a "corrective experience." Hoping someone would see me as a daughter, student, employee who deserved their respect even if they were attracted to me.

It felt like somewhere along the way, I unintentionally became a sorceress, conjuring the worst in people. I knew I wanted attention and affection, and that when I got it, it felt powerful. But the power would always flip. I would find myself backed into a corner I didn't want to be in. It made me feel like I had tainted chemistry, pheromones that called to predators—or potential predators who needed a willing participant. I couldn't understand how this kept happening. *Are these the only relationships I can have with men?*

I later came to understand this as traumatic reenactment. I was compulsively repeating this same pattern with the hope of healing my past. Pulled into the same beginning over and over looking for a different ending. When I received attention from these (often married) men, I felt the familiar pull to try and make it last, to get what I could while I was in their good graces. I eventually played into the sexual dynamic of it all because I could tell that was what they wanted. I couldn't play into the overt sexuality as a

132

child with Randy, but once I became a woman, I knew it was the most effective way to keep their interest. And their interest felt like survival. Like I didn't exist without it.

17

I Can't Stop

Toxic relationships weren't the only pattern that came with me to New York. The further away I got from home, the less I had to prove I wasn't "like them" with regards to my parents' alcoholism. It wasn't long before I was drinking almost daily, listening to sad love songs on my boom box.

I would often wake up on my living room floor next to a puddle of melted candle wax after the flame had burned down to nothing. Or be roused from the smell of charred pots on the stove, burned to a crisp when I had forgotten I'd been cooking spaghetti. It's a miracle my apartment never went up in flames.

My drinking started to impact my ability to pursue music, my entire reason for moving to New York. I would go to bars that had live music and ask if I could sit in for a song. Lead singers would say, "Sure, but not till the last set." This meant many hours later, and for me, many drinks. I could never wait that long to start drinking, and once I started, I couldn't stop. By the time I was asked on stage, I couldn't remember lyrics to songs I had sung a million times.

The same thing happened with auditions. I would have a drink to take the edge off, but one lowered my resistance to the next. Many times, I never even showed up. I would wake up the next day feeling ashamed of myself, like a fraud and a failure.

I sought out a low-cost therapist, but never wanted to talk about my drinking. Every time she asked, I drastically reduced the amount to what seemed appropriate for a young lady. "That seems like a bit much for a social drinker," she replied. Even my lies were drunk.

I started smoking more pot thinking I would drink less, but switching one substance for another never worked. I later declared, "I'm quitting drinking, smoking pot, and cigarettes. I am going to start running, losing weight, and eating healthy!" But I never made it more than a few days. It was so much easier to fail in secret.

One night, I fell down the stairs of whatever bar I'd landed in. Covered in spilled beer and ashes, I squeezed into the women's bathroom between what seemed like hundreds of other girls vying for their own attention in the mirror.

Through my intoxication, my reflection became sharp and penetrating. The room stopped spinning for a moment and I could really see myself. My lack of balance, my lipstick that was trying too hard, the glazed-over eyes I'd had contempt for my entire life. *What are you doing, Ingrid?* I wasn't sure how I was getting home or what happened to the people I called friends earlier that evening.

I finally recognized I needed help. Largely from a phone call from Mita who told me *she* was getting help. I heard her tell me about her own drinking, how bad it'd gotten, and then initially responded with something like, "I'm so proud of you," in a tone that couldn't help but carry a little superiority as avoidance.

But I heard the clarity in her voice when she said, "Asking for help was the best thing I've ever done." I wanted to know that feeling. I wanted to be scooped up and out of the mess I was in, carried to help and safety. So, I stepped up to the plate one more time. I called my parents.

I thought I needed rehab, because that's what Mita needed. I didn't think my dad and Alice had the money, so I called my mom and Randy. When Randy answered, I knew he was the decision maker, so I told him pretty plainly, "I can't stop drinking and I think I need help."

Randy's reply was more consistent than I could have ever imagined. "You just have to become a functional alcoholic like the rest of us."

The fact that he admitted to being an alcoholic stunned me. I'd never heard him say the word in relation to himself. All I could think was, *How can I pretend this was helpful so I can get off the phone?*

The following Monday, I went to my temp job and opened up the phone book looking for help. "A" for alcohol seemed like a good place to start, and I called AA.

"Central Office," a nice man answered.

I was trying to get some general information about how to stop drinking, but Mr. Clairvoyant told me there was a 6:30 meeting around the corner that night and lots of young people would be there. Despite the fact I had turned twenty-one just days before, I was insulted by his insinuation I would be comfortable with *young people*. Young was a dirty word. I was clearly having a midlife crisis. I also knew I wasn't ready to see anyone face to face, but he persisted. So, I left work that night and went to my first meeting.

Crossing the threshold of that doorway was like entering a movie set packed with people who all seemed to have a purpose, buying books, taking pamphlets, and finding their seats. We were downstairs in a brownstone building, occupying the entire bottom floor. Two small rooms and one tiny bathroom were split by a hallway and everywhere I looked had a vintage, yellow hue. I was able to blend in without anyone noticing how much my skin was crawling.

I made my way to a cold, metal folding chair against the brick wall in the back room. To keep myself distracted, I read every piece of "art" on the walls— black frames containing printer paper in an array of colors with sayings like, "Let Go, Let God" and "One day at a time."

Eventually, the man running the meeting started knocking on the folding table. He stood at the front of the room in a suit and tie and asked if anyone was attending for the first time.

I had no intention of raising my hand. But then a girl sitting right next to me raised hers. Admitting she was there for the first time made me feel like I was doing something "wrong" if I didn't do the same. So, I raised my hand just level with my shoulder. When the leader acknowledged me, I said, "My name is Ingrid and I'm not sure if I belong here." *I do not want to belong here.*

The hardest thing about getting sober was admitting I was one of them. That I had become the very thing I was running from and railing against my entire life. I had one true mission: to remain in contempt of my parents' destructive behaviors and prove I was better than them. Now I knew I wasn't, and it felt like a death sentence.

The meeting continued, and one woman's comment stood out more than any other: "People who don't belong in these rooms don't often find themselves here, wondering if they do." *Point taken.* But I still ran for the door when the meeting was over. When I crossed back over that threshold, tears that had been locked up for ages started rushing towards the floodgates.

I was crying so hard I couldn't get on the subway. The close quarters would have suffocated me, so I just kept walking. I started at 37th Street on the east side, and when I had crossed the width of Manhattan, I headed north and wound up in Times Square, the neon lights and hurrying people making it seem like I was walking in slow-motion.

All the feelings I had been trying to numb with alcohol since I was thirteen were welling up to the surface and I had no ability to hold them back. Memory after memory flooded my consciousness. Almost like a movie strip, I saw each fragment of my life, but they were different somehow. It was as though I was being transformed on a cellular level, one frame at a time, in rapid-fire succession. Broken pieces of me were being filled in. Feeling the depth of my pain brought the possibility of healing it. Half of this new reality felt like it would kill me, but the other half felt like it was saving my life.

Seventeen days after I became a legal drinker, I took my last drink. I may have been an alcoholic, but at twenty-one years old, I discovered I could be a sober one. Although I was hoping my sobriety was a finish line of sorts, I eventually found it to be more of a foundation. Something that was necessary if I was to restore an even fuller, stronger self.

18

The Truth is More Interesting

When I went to my second meeting, on my second day of sobriety, I realized people were going to say really invasive things like, "Hi, Ingrid, how are you?" The sound of my own voice was foreign and frightening. Genuine curiosity felt like an interrogation and I didn't know how to share common pleasantries. All of the pressure made me want to drink.

How's this going to work? I needed the meetings, but I absolutely could not talk to anyone about it. So, for the next eighty-eight days, I went to a different meeting every single day, somewhere in the greater boroughs of Manhattan and the Bronx.

On my eighty-ninth day of sobriety, the options were getting thin, so I ventured to a 7:30 a.m. meeting, three subway rides away. As I arrived in the small room, I surprisingly felt more comfortable than I had in a very long time.

The tiny meeting felt like a representation of the entire city. There was the Wall Street tycoon and the veterans living at the VA. There were old and young, black and white, men and women. We definitely represented the notion of "a group that normally would not mix." And yet, there we were, and I finally wanted to go back to the same meeting twice.

The next day happened to be my ninetieth, the day you receive a medallion. Not your average plastic coin saying, "One day at a time," but a metal marker of a significant event in sobriety. It had weight to it, metaphorically and otherwise.

Several group members asked if I would return the next day so I could celebrate with them. I had every intention to and was excited, but the following morning, I slept through my alarm. I was so accustomed to steep punishments for honest mistakes, I figured this would be no different. *This is so fucked up, now I can never go back.*

I was full of self-loathing as I made my way to the subway station that cold December morning in the Bronx. It was freezing outside as I approached the outdoor, cement stairs that often iced over after a storm. And on this day, my ninetieth day of sobriety, there was an elderly woman sitting in the middle of the walkway, waiting for someone to help her down. I was barely able to see her through my self-pity, but arm-in-arm, I helped her to the station.

Later that day, I shared with my sponsor Lori about the magical meeting I had been to the day before and how I was certain I'd failed them and in turn, failed myself. "The only way I can go back is if I tell them there was a natural disaster or power outage that turned off my alarm." I figured if it wasn't my fault, maybe they could forgive me.

Lori's answer was profound: "Ingrid, the truth is much more interesting than the lie. You were so excited to go back to the same meeting, to celebrate ninety days, you couldn't sleep last night. You slept through your alarm because you were exhausted and God had other plans for you this morning. You were meant to help that woman down the stairs."

I knew she was right. I immediately felt sad for all of the times I'd told lies, people-pleasing lies, in an effort to get people to see me, or like me, or forgive me. Suddenly, the truth was not only easier, it was a richer, fuller telling of what happened. It allowed me to like myself. And Lori wasn't put off by my truth, she wasn't using it to manipulate or judge me. She was using it to get to know me better and to help me grow. It was such a relief.

I went back to the morning meeting on day ninety-one. One man said he'd brought me flowers the day before, and it practically shattered me. But when it was my turn to share, I said how meaningful it was that they were so welcoming, how grateful I was I didn't have to keep running, even from one meeting to the next. I told them I wanted to lie, to make it not my fault so they wouldn't hate me, but I wanted to tell the truth even more.

I went back to that meeting on day ninety-two and ninety-three and every day there was a meeting in that room for the rest of my first year of sobriety. They became my "home group" and the members definitely became my family of choice as I began to tolerate being seen and heard from people who wanted to see and hear me. We would all go to the diner across the street after the meeting for breakfast. When I shared that I had booked a gig as a singer/songwriter at The Bitter End, half the group showed up to the front row of my show, cheering me on with wide smiles as I sang, one hundred percent present and sober. I was finally able to show up for what I wanted, with conscious effort, continuity and real support.

The one and only time I considered relapse, I was sitting in a nondescript cubicle, in a high-rise somewhere in Manhattan. I'd hidden a one-pound bag of peanut M&Ms in my desk drawer, hoping they would provide some comfort as painful feelings were welling up.

I stepped outside for lunch and realized I left the M&Ms upstairs. I wanted them, but I couldn't go back to get them. I couldn't go back at all and I never did. This was unlike me; I had become reliable to a fault.

I ended up walking to Grand Central Station, awash in miserable memories about Randy that left me disoriented. Feeling so lost in a place designed to take you somewhere amplified my confusion. I didn't know where to go or how to get there. My thoughts were fueled by self-hatred and I was certain this sobriety business was bullshit. *Nothing is going to change my past. Nothing can re-write everything that's happened.* I felt like I would never be free of my torment, the worthlessness I had been carrying for so long. I was just left to *feel* it all now, and it was excruciating.

I looked up and saw the majestically painted ceiling in Grand Central. It's covered with the constellations, seemingly guiding the millions of visitors below. I found myself ushered towards the payphones that hung in a large circle, off to the side of the room. The bustle and noise gave me no personal space, and yet it also helped me to feel invisible in the throngs of the faceless people around me.

I pulled a quarter from my pocket and called Lori. This was something we were told to do: "Always carry change and if you want to pick up a drink, pick up the phone instead." Despite her busy life working for the corporate office of a major fashion house, Lori answered. I was always astounded at the time she freely gave me.

I wanted to thank her for everything she'd done, and then tell her goodbye. "I'm sorry, but I don't think I can do this," I said. I was pressing the receiver against my face, leaning deep into the payphone bank so I could hear her soft-spoken voice. My own voice was buried in tears and apologies.

She asked if I had my "big book" (the basic text of AA) with me. I happened to have a copy in the large, leather backpack I was carrying. Lori asked me to take it out, and although I didn't want to be seen with it in public, I removed it from my bag. I opened the book to the page she referenced and then read a passage out loud. My willingness surpassed my embarrassment as I recited the words.

"No matter how far down the scale we have gone...." I took a pause. No matter how bad things used to be, no matter how "bad" I thought I was, this phrase seemed to imply some hope. Maybe I couldn't understand any of this, but Lori was encouraging me to hang in there because *she* believed, and *the book* believed I could have a new experience. Maybe I could believe that too.

It was enough for me not to pick up a drink that day.

One day during that first year, a homeless man walked into our meeting after it started. He was visibly drunk, talking to himself, and I found it upsetting. I imagined it was upsetting to others and I looked over to the "old-timer" sitting next to me. He whispered, "If he was able to stop drinking on his own, he wouldn't need to be here with us."

The permission given to that man, to be exactly who he was, as he was, was astounding. My need to be "perfect," even in a meeting full of drunks, softened for a moment when I heard such acceptance and compassion. We were all just people, wounded people who couldn't stop drinking without the help of one another. I thought back to my short time in that Christian church, how I never felt good enough to belong. It was comforting to find a sense of belonging in the opposite of "good," by admitting my brokenness, in church basements throughout the city.

19

Internal Straitjacket

When I'd been living in New York for three years, my trio was playing gigs all over the city. But I wasn't making any money with music. I realized I needed to learn how to sight-read if I wanted to audition as a backup singer or record commercials. So, I revamped my high school dream of going to Berklee College of Music in Boston.

I began the application process and soon discovered I wouldn't qualify for financial aid without my parents' tax returns. Students younger than twenty-four were still seen as minors in the government's eyes, which made me so mad. I had been on my own for six years. I hated that I had to get "permission" from my mom and Randy to go back to school, but that's what I had to do. I decided to talk with them on a trip to Colorado.

On the first morning of my visit, I was standing in the kitchen with my mom, trying to get her attention. "Mom … Mom … Hellooo?!" She was three feet away from me in their designer log cabin but was clearly lost in another world.

When she finally snapped back into her body, we had one of the most honest moments of our relationship. "Ingrid, sometimes my life is so painful I just have to disappear for a little while."

I stopped breathing and could have choked on my tears. "I know it is, Mom. I know it is."

I would have leaned over to give her a hug, but I didn't want to invite self-consciousness into the moment or for her to pull herself together like I'd seen so many times. I stared at my mom, motionless as Randy came in to make his favorite skillet breakfast, asking how everyone would like their eggs.

"Over hard," I said, feeling heartbroken about the truth my mom had just shared. But I was grateful she shared it. It was a rare moment of real intimacy between us. And now it was gone.

I waited until the evening to bring up Berklee and was trying to get them excited about the idea. "I want to go back to college and seriously pursue being a musician." I didn't think my request of their taxes was that big of a deal. I wasn't asking them to pay for school, just to give me some information so I could get the loans to pay for it myself.

"It's nobody's business how much money I make," Randy said, shutting the conversation down quickly.

I tried shifting it to my mom. "But Mom, I can't get loans unless you give me your taxes. Are you literally going to block me from going to school?"

As usual, she didn't say a word. It all felt like punishment for not taking the deal Randy offered me years earlier. I was so mad and left our dinner to sulk in their guest bedroom, wishing we weren't so far from the Denver airport.

I was in the kitchen the next morning when Randy asked to speak with me. I finished making my cup of orange cappuccino, the instant coffee my mom had loved since I was a little girl, then joined him at the kitchen table. We were surrounded by picture windows and bright mountain sunlight. The idyllic setting was trying to penetrate the knot in my stomach.

"I won't give you my taxes," he said. "But I will pay for Berklee."

Okay, here we go again.

I waited for him to explain the catch and he didn't disappoint. Randy said he would pay for school, but not my living expenses. Of course, I knew his son John was currently attending Berklee as a drummer and that Randy was paying for his tuition *and* living expenses. Giving me some, but not all, the money I needed felt worse than him not giving me their tax returns. I would have been happier assuming the debt.

"I appreciate the offer, but I wasn't asking you to pay for school. This is something I want to do on my own," I said.

"Well, this is the only way I'm going to help. You can take it or leave it."

I looked down at my coffee, resting on the dining table of my childhood. It felt as though the ornate legs of the wooden base had wrapped themselves around my limbs. I looked up just past Randy and was almost shocked to see my twenty-three-year-old self in the mirrored China cabinet, a more grownup version of the girl being held hostage at the table.

"Let me think about it," I said before walking outside. I made my way to the swing perched in the middle of the grass. I tried swinging, but I felt like I was wearing an internal straitjacket. You couldn't see it on the outside, but it was perfectly fastened just under my skin. If ever I was able to wrestle a little freedom, if I was finding ease, comfort, or success, it made Randy uncomfortable and he'd tighten the straps. I could have swung for hours, I could have disappeared into another world like my mom, but it wouldn't loosen the squeeze.

Later that day, I sat with my mom on the porch outside her bedroom. She took a deep drag on her cigarette and blew smoke far out in front of us before she said, "Ingrid, take this offer. It's the only way you'll be able to go to school."

Although it killed part of the excitement I was feeling, I knew she was right. I knew she was trying to encourage me from the constraints of her own straitjacket. Like she was saying, *just take his money*, and I appreciated the permission. It shifted the focus from what I wasn't getting, to what I was. We were silently agreeing that tuition was a perk for putting up with so much shit. I went back to New York and finished my application.

When I was accepted to Berklee, I moved to Boston and lived with my stepbrother John and his friend. Randy had been paying John's half of the rent, but now it was divided into three, and I had to get temp jobs to send Randy my portion.

I tried to feel grateful for the tuition, but sending Randy that check every month while he gave John everything felt terrible. It was manageable on a practical level, but it wasn't emotionally sustainable. It was a monthly tether to his punishment and control.

After singing in Berklee's prestigious gospel choir, even singing back up for L.L. Cool J at the Fleet Center one night, I only stayed at Berklee for one year.

I had met an exchange student from The Rotterdam Conservatory in Holland and learned it was ten percent of Berklee's tuition. The Dutch would also give me a grant as a student from outside the European Union, and they didn't need tax returns for the rest. In some ways, it felt more prestigious than Berklee, you had to audition to get in. *Excuse me while I try on these wooden clogs.*

I was twenty-four with freshly cut bangs, waiting in the hall for my audition. When it was my turn, I walked inside and gave my music to the pianist. I was incredibly nervous but felt my confidence rise as my bluesy voice filled the cavernous room. When I was done, I looked at the panel of judges, ready to excuse myself while they discussed things in private. But they gave a quick glance to one another and told me I didn't have to leave. I was offered acceptance on the spot.

I was elated. I moved to The Netherlands and rode my vintage bike through the streets. I joined several bands, singing in cafes all over the country. I fell in love with the Dutch people, who all seemed so kind, generous, and a foot taller than me. I stayed sober by attending the one English-speaking meeting in Rotterdam. Every Wednesday night there were usually four or five expats, rolling our own cigarettes and drinking tiny cups of coffee.

But after one year, I decided to move back to the States. I knew that's where I needed to establish a career and although I had never been to Los Angeles, I thought that was the next best place to pursue my goals.

So, I set off for another clean slate. I loved the idea of starting fresh, where everything felt possible. Where I felt *brand new*. I started another band, wrote more music and performed all over LA. But after a couple more years, my passion felt like an expensive hobby. I still loved singing, but I was tired of being someone's secretary to support it. I knew I would always be an artist, but I was heading toward thirty and wanted to drop the "starving" adjective.

When I thought about what I'd like to do if I wasn't going to be a singer, there was only one answer. I wanted to help people. I wanted to really *know* people. Lori and I still talked all the time, but the longer I was gone from New York, the more we thought I should work with someone local. My new sponsor in LA was in the mental health field and could see how interested I was. She suggested I might go back to school to finish the degree in psychology I started at Colorado State.

Maybe the little girl in me, the one who was hunting for answers as a child, could finally find some. Maybe I could be there for others the way my sponsors and AA community had been there for me. And perhaps I might even be there for people in the ways I had been overlooked, the ways I would remain overlooked for many more years. Although I came to sit on numerous therapist's couches, trying to sort out what still haunted me, no one seemed to get to the root of my pain. There was something missing in my journey towards wholeness and I was desperate to find it.

20

"Real Trauma"

It took me twelve years and five schools, but I finally finished my bachelor's degree. It was now 2004, I was twenty-nine and well into my Masters in psychology, loving the process of learning and hoping to become a licensed psychotherapist.

One afternoon on a Malibu hillside, I was attending a training at the dual-diagnosis treatment center where I had an internship. Dr. Bessel van der Kolk, a renowned psychiatrist and leader in the field of traumatic stress, was sharing a case study when I experienced time starting to slow. My mouth became sticky and dry, my heart beat like a kettle drum. Surrounded by twenty other clinicians, I imagined sliding into the crease of my chair, the incredible shrinking therapist.

I had never experienced a natural disaster, lived through a war or life-threatening car crash, so I never categorized my own experiences as *"real trauma."* I would have been ashamed if anyone knew I was considering the label as personal to me. But as I learned about childhood trauma, what he called *developmental trauma*, without overly clinical language, I held back a cry that could have overtaken the room.

Dr. van der Kolk shared about his patient, a young woman who came from an alcoholic home where she experienced covert sexual abuse. She became an alcoholic herself and vacillated between disassociation and hypervigilance. "It was too painful for this woman to inhabit her own body," he said with his strong Dutch accent. "Can you imagine this type of psychic pain?"

I was not inhabiting my body as I watched him pace the room, eventually standing directly by my side. *He was telling my story.* I looked up at Dr. van der Kolk from my chair and he seemed like a giant. A friendly, towering giant. I could feel his compassion, the way he seemed to care for the woman he had been treating. He wanted us to understand the complexity of her symptoms: her depression, addictions, impulsivity, and acting out sexually were all an outgrowth of pervasive, childhood trauma.

At that point in my life, it had become easy to talk about my alcoholism. I was proud of my recovery. But all the ways I still didn't like or trust myself, all the ways I still felt broken were shrouded in shame.

Learning how wounding in childhood could lead to post-traumatic stress disorder (PTSD)—a switch was flipped in my brain. I went from someone with a story to someone who had actual pain for actual reasons. With Dr. van der Kolk's seeming permission, I was starting to make sense to myself. *These are trauma responses.*

He went on to discuss how secrecy often plays a role in childhood trauma. The combination of being hurt, without a compassionate witness, can lead someone to feel as though they are fundamentally flawed.

How often had I thought, *it wasn't that bad,* while judging myself for being haunted by my past? No matter where I moved or what I accomplished, all roads led back to my chasm of confusion. *Did I make the whole thing up? Why is every waking thought tied to Randy?* Exposing the fact that I was relating to these case presentations would have exposed these questions, and I wasn't ready. It felt too risky.

I believed my alcoholism could help me work with other addicts, because I was on the "other side" of addiction and in recovery. I was nine-years sober. But this was an area I had no recovery in at all. I needed to believe, and I needed the people in that room to believe, that my past wasn't still defining me. Owning that truth, even to myself, felt like I had failed, like I had no business trying to be of service to people who were genuinely suffering.

So, I remained in limbo. A part of me knew I experienced trauma, in a colloquial sense at least, and perhaps I identified with some aspects of PTSD. But the other part—the part that wasn't taken care of as a child, who was called a liar—maintained an allegiance to my parents' side of the story.

All their gaslighting, the way they manipulated the truth and blamed me for my pain, had taken root. I internalized their lies and began to self-gaslight. I believed I was the problem. I believed I deserved to feel ashamed for not "getting over it by now." Getting over it was my salvation, and it could only happen by my parents' admission of the truth, or through my own rising above it.

I tried to get over it with therapy. I really wanted to feel freer, in my skin and in my life. It felt like I told my story hundreds of times. I never suppressed it and I knew my experience with Randy was wrong. I just didn't trust that his intentions were as bad as I originally suspected. And I didn't think my suffering was warranted if I hadn't experienced more obvious violations. I didn't know what I experienced was *traumatic*, and what that meant from a physiological standpoint.

I couldn't draw a line from my past to my current expression of symptoms, so I called them by another name. I mostly thought I had anxiety—which can mean a lot of different things, but for me, it meant living in a perpetual state of walking on eggshells, constantly scanning for threats, particularly in relationships.

I was constantly afraid of "getting in trouble," or someone being mad at me—habitually guarding against these unfounded fears by overcompensating. No matter my age or how long it had been since I lived at home, if I experienced a small conflict, my body felt like a lockdown was coming.

I talked about these fears with my therapists, and mostly felt embarrassed. Like, I knew it sounded ridiculous, so I should let it go. Logically, my colleague didn't suddenly hate me. When I said as much in therapy, it was as though the intellectual understanding was sufficient. Intellectualizing was perceived as "insight," which seemed synonymous with wellness. But it never removed the *feelings*. The feelings were real and dictating my responses. I was overwhelmed and couldn't shake it. I felt like I was doomed. The constant stress brought on physical symptoms like chronic migraine attacks, psoriasis and shingles.

While Dr. van der Kolk opened a door for me to understand trauma in a more complex way, I couldn't get past my minimization. None of my therapists helped me get past it either. When I secretly looked more closely at the diagnostic criteria for PTSD, I didn't think I qualified for a diagnosis because I never had a flashback. I thought they were all like the ones we see in the movies, with a specific memory, strong visual and auditory component. Like a veteran who hears a car backfire on the street and is suddenly back in active combat.

Many years later, I learned that flashbacks are defined as *any* way we reexperience our traumatic past as though it's happening right now. Most of my therapy sessions throughout my life were one long recitation of whatever manifestation of trauma I was experiencing at the time. I just didn't know it because the flashbacks weren't tied to a specific memory. They felt solely related to a current event. They just felt "real." *I am bad, I am a loser, everything is about to fall apart.*

In all my years of sitting on therapist's couches, I never knew I needed to work with a trauma therapist. I didn't know how to ask a therapist what they specialized in at all. I just looked up "therapist" and showed up, like whomever held that title was holding all the answers. And working with therapists who didn't understand trauma meant they couldn't help me make these connections. They couldn't give me accurate language for my life because they saw it through a different lens.

Telling my story over and over with people who couldn't comprehend it was like weeding a garden with kitchen scissors. Cutting off the leaves while the roots kept branching underground. I didn't understand that trauma is stored in the body, in a pre-verbal, primitive way. Recovery often needs to happen through deeper, experiential modes of healing. Traditional talk therapy, aimed at insight and compassion, doesn't work directly with the nervous system—the part of us that is most impacted. The logical mind carries a different understanding to our lived and learned experience. They speak a different language.

And then there's the fact I was doing all this "work" in therapy, while I maintained relationships with the people who had hurt me, like nothing ever happened. I continually privileged my parents' denial just to be in my family. As a result, every time I called home, interacted with Randy, experienced myself as "the problem"... every time my mom didn't show up for me, protect me, or know me at all, it reinforced the original wounds.

All the selfcare loaded on one side of the scale was counteracted by engaging with the same people in the same ways, even if the engagement was limited. I unknowingly condoned their behavior and reinforced my pain by shoving it below the surface. In order to stay in relationship, I abandoned myself and my body was listening: *I am unworthy. I don't deserve love. Dysfunction is relationship.*

I never knew I had PTSD, or the later understanding of Complex PTSD (CPTSD). I remained in constant management of myself, always striving and never healing. It's like I knew I had a disorder but no one gave me an accurate diagnosis, which made me think it was just *me*. My therapists ended up colluding with the idea that I was the problem by suggesting I do *this* or *that* differently related to anxiety or depression. Without seeing my symptoms in context, they stayed in constant rotation, like a whack-a-mole game.

I spent the next decade doing the same dance as before: striving for external successes that might make me feel whole, while simultaneously feeling unworthy. It was always up to something or someone *out there* to fix me. And if it was always out there, it was never in *here*. Not in this moment. Not within me.

My striving for approval never felt like a choice. It felt like survival. My "enoughness" was always on the line. *Can I achieve enough to finally feel safe in the world?* It felt like I needed something big to arrest my anxieties, my perfectionism, and my *Ingridness*.

Dr. van der Kolk opened a door for me that day, but it wasn't one I could walk through. I was on fierce auto-pilot, passing for someone who belonged in that armchair. I was leaning into my newfound credentials and hating the version of me who could have been a patient. My particulars never deserved the kind of care and attention van der Kolk was offering. So, the thing that could have helped me recover from trauma— facing my shame and believing I had experienced trauma—was also a trigger.

I already knew what happened when I faced my past head-on with my family: it blew up in my face. It made things worse. The part of me who was living in survival mode was never going to let that happen again. I would do whatever it took to find another way forward, one that didn't involve facing that kind of vulnerability, ever again.

21

The Red Face

Halfway through my master's degree, I decided to pursue a PhD in psychology. My subconscious plan was to get to a place where "old Ingrid" no longer existed. Surely a doctorate would give me some solid ground to stand on, some assurance I had finally arrived.

I was also genuinely curious if I had the capacity to get a PhD. Could I really go from "Ding" to "Doctor?" I still didn't see myself as "smart," but I was often looking for the edges of a thing, so I could see myself in relation to it. Looking for anything to reflect my true self because I still didn't know who she was.

I pursued things where my perfectionism felt like an asset, where I could push myself towards a clear and achievable goal. Operation Constant Striving was in full effect and it was propelling me forward at a rapid pace. But it also left me exposed, giving opportunity for the *red face* to surface. The red face was external evidence of my lack of self-esteem, all the ways I thought I was flawed. It was beyond my control and would leak out as a reminder of who I still was on the inside.

I may have been perfectly fine moving to a big city by myself, even to a new country, but going to a fancy grocery store in my twenties was incredibly intimidating (okay, maybe it still is). You know the ones, with all the organic fruit and milk that costs twice as much? In an upscale neighborhood where the residents evidently deserve better? I had such little self-worth I would practically break out in hives when I tried shopping in these stores.

I was so ashamed of my inferior wardrobe or making a sound in the soup aisle, my face turned bright red. The experience was dreadful, and yet it was sure to capture me on these outings and other less predictable ones. If I were talking to someone I admired and they asked me a question, any question really, my face would turn crimson as they awaited my reply. Not in a cute, blushing sort of way. We're talking volcano red, and I would start profusely sweating.

One day, at work in Los Angeles as an administrative assistant, I was sitting at my desk when my boss came back from lunch with a friend. He was confident, successful and well dressed. Standing above the partition that divided us, he and his handsome friend were feeling chatty and asked what I had done for lunch.

I had just finished a Lean Cuisine for one, in my cubicle. *How am I going to tell them that? "Yeah, lunch with friends sounds great, but I prefer cheese cannelloni in a microwavable bowl."* Once I felt the red face coming on, I was sure they saw it too, and that's when things got really out of hand. I had to pretend the red face wasn't there while grasping for something that passed for normal dialogue.

So, when I went back to school for psychology, I wanted to know all the material before my first class. If I already knew everything, I wouldn't make an ass out of myself. But then how was I ever to learn? School was the place to do it, so I had to face my shame.

I wanted to participate in class. I wanted to engage with my peers, so school became my own version of exposure therapy: confronting my fears one red face at a time. I eventually learned to tolerate the anxious, sweaty feeling until it largely went away. As I got more accustomed to *being seen*, I became less ashamed. It was like being visible in the world had been another trigger. Asking a question in class was basically asking for help, and it was terrifying—so my toxic shame—the belief that I was worthless, rushed through my whole body.

I didn't see this as a trauma response at the time. I only saw the red face as an enormous defect, something I didn't see "regular people" like my classmates experiencing.

Pushing myself towards betterment, I completed my coursework, clinical training and dissertation all within four years—one of only two people in my cohort to complete the program in such a short period of time.

The day I realized what I'd accomplished wasn't when I defended my dissertation or crossed the stage to receive my degree. It was weeks later at a Korean spa in Los Angeles.

I made an appointment for a Korean scrub, a ritual where you lay naked on a massage table while a masseur exfoliates every inch of your body with a coarse mitt. It's an oddly painful and relaxing experience. I felt like a baby with no motor control, receiving my first bath.

The awkwardness eventually gives way to a sense of freedom. Even the vulnerability of being naked fades into the background. All shame about my body disappeared in the face of being stripped down on every level. There was no hiding, covering or pretending, just the experience itself as layers of dead skin fell away.

After the treatment, the masseur delivered me to the sauna. The spa was busy that day, but I was alone in what felt like a sacred space. The sound of the cedar bench creaking beneath my weight reminded me of early childhood. My Finnish grandmother had a sauna and I used to love throwing water on the hot rocks, watching the steam sizzle and rise.

The smell in this sauna was just the same, sweet but almost too hot to breathe through my nose. Staring at the hourglass filled with pink sand, I began silently reflecting on everything that led up to this moment. As the heat penetrated my bones, a wave of emotion came over me. I said out loud in the dimly lit room, "I did it. I really did it." And then I started to sob.

As my hungry pores absorbed the steam, a truth was landing in my body for the first time. *I'm not stupid.* I don't recall if I said those words out loud, but I heard them. And I believed it. If this was the only thing I got from those three letters after my name, I would have happily done it all again.

I knew it wasn't just a degree or knowledge I had gained, it was a reconnection to my sense of *knowing*. Finding the edge of the thing allowed me to feel the capacity I had all along. My parents made me doubt my own intelligence, but I would never doubt it again. That was the moment I knew I graduated, buck-naked, all alone on a cedar bench. Red-faced in a rosy cheek kind of way.

22

Red Flags

By the time I turned thirty, I had been through so many unhealthy relationships, I wondered if I would ever get married. Time and again, I dated men who weren't right for me, who told me in one way or another they didn't want a commitment. I seemed particularly drawn to liars, cheaters, and active alcoholics—each time trying to convince them to stay with me until they broke things off.

But Mark and I seemed to want the same things for our future: kids, travel, an idyllic life. We met through an online dating site when I'd moved to the Bay Area for graduate school and he lived in LA. The distance wasn't ideal, but we both jumped in through long emails and phone calls into the night. He was Hollywood handsome in his pictures, six feet tall with brown hair and blue eyes. I fell in love with him before we ever met in person.

When we finally met, six weeks later, I knew deep down he wasn't right for me. But I wasn't able to listen to that feeling. I had never heard the saying: Red flags don't look like red flags when they feel like home. I didn't know I couldn't even *see* red flags—and that was the biggest red flag of all. The truth is they were all there on the first date.

I had driven to LA and wore my new, low-rise Seven jeans and a tight-fitting top. Knowing Mark had almost a foot on me, I wore five-inch platform sandals.

His apartment was tucked into the corner of a huge building in the San Fernando Valley. I wound my way through the labyrinth and knocked. *Thank God!* I thought. He looked just like his pictures.

He invited me in and I looked around. "What's going on with all the sheets?" I asked. Half of the living room and what I could see of the bedroom were draped in linens.

"Oh, this is an apartment my friend and I rented when we were shooting our movie. We needed a place for colleagues to stay."

Mark never mentioned he was staying in a spare apartment. *Where was his place? What was he doing here now?*

I didn't ask these questions. Instead, I immediately pivoted to the more pleasant details of his story: he had rented this apartment to host industry professionals for the movie he had produced. He was aware that the place was sort of a dump, with tacky furnishings, he'd never want to *live* in a place like that.

These first fifteen minutes could have told me so much, but I embellished his inventions with my own magic touches. I didn't want to see the sheets as a sign he was hiding something. I showed up to our first date with a suitcase and every intention of staying for the weekend.

We made our way to the couch and it was awkward talking in person after only speaking on the phone. I wanted to look anywhere but at him. I'm not sure how we got to the subject, but he was suddenly sharing that he'd once had a problem with drinking. It seemed he was trying to emphasize our similarities and compatibility, but my gut told me something else.

It wasn't just that he could have a few too many cocktails. Mark had gone to the hospital after living in a drunken stupor for days. I wasn't clear about the timeline, but it seemed recent. *He knows I'm sober, why didn't he tell me this before?*

"I didn't realize you had a problem with drinking," I said. "I'm really sorry to hear about it, but I'm surprised you didn't share this earlier." I tried to be honest.

I watched as Mark began to backpedal. He seemed confused as to why I wasn't applauding his honesty. My obvious apprehension was making him mad.

"I just told you something I've never told anyone and you're making it all about *you*," he said.

My body heard him say, *You are so selfish!*

"Besides, I'm totally fine now. That was a long time ago. I haven't had a drink in over a year and don't plan on it anytime soon," he continued.

I went from being somewhat discerning, to shutting down completely. I left my body sitting next to him on the couch and wanted to change the subject as badly as he did. Somehow, we decided it was time to leave for dinner and we focused on that.

Staring out the car window, the vibration of the road was like a peace offering to my frightened system: *Come on back, it's okay.* As we pulled into the valet, I began to recognize something more congruent with the relationship Mark and I had created over the phone. We were shown to a cozy booth in the Italian restaurant, and it finally felt good to be in his presence. He smelled nice and was complimentary. We talked for hours like we'd done before, only now we were snuggled up next to each other. We laughed until we were the last customers in the restaurant.

The check had been sitting on our table for a bit when Mark picked it up. "I'll get it this time because you drove so far," he said. I found the disclaimer jarring and almost offered to pay. But I was trying to break the habit of compulsive caretaking and found myself saying, "Okay, thanks."

We continued dating long-distance and whenever something bothered me, I attempted to bring it up, but the same pattern unfolded. Mark deflected my concerns by talking about our "great love," or by making things my fault. They both had the effect of silencing me. I was desperate for us to move in together, as though that would fix what wasn't working and give us more time to enjoy what was.

When Mark agreed to move in, I had this funny feeling, like we were playing house. Not in a, *this is new and exciting* kind of way but in a, *I am pretending this is real* kind of way. Particularly when he stopped contributing to our bills and I had to pay our overhead with my student loans. I didn't mind that he wanted to be an actor, but I wanted him to get a job to support it like I'd always done with my music.

We once opened a joint savings account, for our future trip to Italy, but one day I discovered he had been withdrawing funds as fast as I deposited them. He claimed he had done nothing wrong and was angry I brought it up in such an accusatory fashion. I felt the only way to move forward was for me to take full responsibility. *Of course, paying his union dues takes priority over Italy, why was I so upset?* I minimized my feelings and his behavior (with his help) until it was no longer a big deal. Problem solved.

I really wanted a family. Mark was the first person I had dated who seemed open to marrying me. So, I kept moving us towards that goal post like my life depended on it. We had been dating for two years when we were visiting Mark's hometown one weekend, walking towards the beach. As we got closer to the water, Mark turned to me and took out a small, silver band from his pocket, "Ingrid, will you marry me?"

It was the moment I was waiting for—pushing for—–but if I were honest with myself, it didn't feel right. I wasn't filled with love and excitement; I was judging his proposal. None of it matched the narrative we'd been working so hard to achieve: *Everything is perfect over here!*

I answered, "Yes," and we kissed as though it was a great love story, but the ring turned my finger green within an hour. It felt like external evidence of our incompatibility, but I focused on the thrill of being engaged. I knew I could fix the ring, make it pretty like I'd done with so many other details. Mark eventually said the band was just temporary and we went ring shopping, quickly finding something we both loved. I turned to him with a huge smile. "Is this the one?" I said, like we were in a commercial for the Shane Company.

Standing in front of the salesman, Mark turned to me. "If you can put it on your credit card, I will make the payments." I didn't see this coming, but I handed my visa over to the salesperson. Though he later repeated his promise to pay for the ring, he never made a single one and neither of us brought it up again.

We were married by an officiant in Central Park, New York with my sponsor Lori and her husband, David, as our witnesses. I felt so happy. Or at least I was hopeful. But shortly after we got back to LA, I began finding parking tickets hiding in my glove box. We eventually couldn't afford our modest apartment, so I found us a cheaper place to live. I hated that he was still choosing not to work but I made the move with enthusiasm. *Look at us taking control of our financial lives!* There was always a kernel of truth in the minimization, but that's what makes every good lie a successful one.

All the while, Mark made us delicious dinners and we enjoyed watching movies on the couch. But this only obscured his lying and manipulating and all the ways I made it my fault.

One afternoon, right before our second wedding anniversary, Mark was in the shower and he and I were fighting through the curtain. I don't remember what we were yelling, but from the safety of his preoccupation, my gut spoke so loudly I couldn't ignore it.

I had never consciously thought about opening our hall closet, but when I did, I saw a suitcase tucked between boxes and boots. I pulled it into the light of the hallway and as I lifted the lid, I saw it was full of empty vodka bottles.

I never realized Mark was passed-out drunk when I got home at night, I thought he was in a "deep sleep." I didn't register the smell of alcohol on his skin because I thought it was his hairspray. I was clean and sober for nine years when we met—I wanted to be a person who wasn't bothered by someone else's drinking. But I certainly was uncomfortable with *alcoholic* drinking. I asked Mark for a separation. I wasn't ready to face a failed marriage, a failed attempt at a successful life, so I gave him a month to move out in the hope he would turn things around.

He didn't. And I finally stopped listening to the hopefulness of his promises and started looking squarely at his actions. I didn't budge on my request for him to go and he eventually moved out.

When I was all alone, without the need to paint a pretty picture or deny what I was experiencing, a funny thing happened. I was literally pinching myself with this Pinocchio feeling, *I'm a real, live boy!* Like admitting the truth was giving me life. And the more real I felt, the more I knew I couldn't go back to the relationship. It wasn't even a choice.

Even though I was certain I'd blown my chance at happiness, that I was a disaster for being a therapist who worked with addiction and had married an active alcoholic … it was incredibly liberating.

For the first time in my life, I stopped waiting for someone to choose me over alcohol. I stopped waiting to be chosen by someone who didn't respect me and I chose myself.

My divorce was the first time I ever broke up with anyone. I'd previously thought I needed to make sense of a potential partner's dysfunction rather than see it as a sign I should leave. I had no real deal breakers because lying and stealing were behaviors to feel sorry for. I simply had to help my partner get the support they needed, so they could stop hurting me and start loving me. I knew intellectually that my relationship patterns went deep into my childhood, but that didn't remove how comfortable I felt with them, their resonance of *home*. "Knowing better" never relieved me of my chemistry and I couldn't force myself into being attracted to a kind and available person.

When I stopped waiting for Mark to see my worth, I finally saw my own pain and loved myself enough to walk away. For so long, I thought if I was the only person who really loved me, it didn't really count. But leaving Mark let me know that my own love is the most important of all. *I had to choose me even though no one else ever did.*

23

It's Okay to Want It

After my divorce from Mark, I went through a grieving period so deep and dark it seemed to stir up all my old demons and bad habits. I started smoking again, secretly, like when I was a teenager living at home. There were many days I didn't want to get out of bed. I knew with every fiber of my being I would never have a family of my own.

I forced myself to meet some friends for breakfast one Saturday and started sharing about my plans to expand my private practice. Now thirty-eight and two years out from my divorce, I was trying to lean into what *was* working in my life: mothering my clients.

There was something alchemical about my job as a therapist; it seemed to not only help my clients, it helped me too. Seeing their humanity always allowed me to soften towards my own. And if that was the only thing going well, I was going to make it as impactful as I could.

Speaking about renting new office space, I spied a little girl twirling in front of the dessert case in the restaurant. She could see her own reflection in the glass and was watching the folds of her pink and yellow skirt whisk up into the air. True joy personified.

While attempting to hold the thread of my thought, outside the corner of my mouth came a quiet and muffled, "That's what I *really* want."

"Wait, what?" My friends stopped short, sensing the direction of our conversation had shifted.

"No, no, no. Let's not go there. Remember how old I am? How single I am? That ship has sailed..." There was humor and heartache in my voice and I couldn't look them in the eyes. I wanted to change the subject. But from across the table came a sincere and kind message, "Ingrid, it's okay to want it."

Tears filled my eyes. I knew they were right. It didn't matter if it felt *possible* to have a family. It was okay that I still wanted it. In fact, I couldn't *not* want it if I tried.

So, I got serious. I've always been at least woo-woo adjacent, drawn to the mystical and magical. I have yet to meet a method of healing I didn't find some value in. I know enough to know that I don't have all the answers, so I sought out an energy worker to cut cords with my past. I made lists of what I wanted and what I would never tolerate again. I read it to my friend and it felt like a shamanic exercise, casting out the bad and creating a foundation for something new.

I realized I felt different as I responded to various dating profiles, like I was done looking for someone to convince or "fix." I wanted an entirely different experience with a partner and the very next person who asked me on a date was Yancey.

He was a year younger than me and had never been married, but included photos of himself and his adorable niece on his profile, so I assumed there was at least some interest in children. We chatted only briefly before he suggested we meet in person.

He chose a nice restaurant and when I arrived, I thought he was more handsome in person, with this wild brown hair that seemed to roam in every direction. We were both a little nervous, but sitting across the table, I realized I was really enjoying our conversation. Yancey was kind, and I experienced an unfamiliar ease in his presence. It felt so effortless, part of me thought, *Maybe we're just meant to be friends.* There was no "all systems go" electric spark like I was used to, but I began to wonder if those sparks were better at announcing insanity than healthy chemistry.

Early in our relationship, we went to the mountains for the fourth of July. "What's the worst that can happen?" we said. "We each read a good book by the lake?"

While we did have quiet moments of solitude, coffees in one hand and a book in the other, we also went on hikes and watched the fireworks. We rented a canoe and lay in the warm sun on the sandy inlet. We ducked into the bedroom between every outdoor adventure and then we'd leisurely make food in the little cabin we rented. It didn't feel like playing house, it felt like the version of home I had always wanted.

I even brought my new Vita-mix blender because we were excited to make smoothies. Not to be outdone by my appliance offering, Yancey brought a rice cooker. *A rice cooker.* He actually *bought* it for the occasion, which delighted me to no end. It was one of the many ways he surprised me and brought me joy.

I had been sober for almost two decades at this point. Yancey wasn't sure what to call his relationship to alcohol, except he had recently decided it wasn't for him. I was initially worried that history was repeating itself but soon came to differentiate between Yancey's honesty and so many others' denial.

My sponsor Bill was immensely helpful, as always, in helping to unpack my confusion. Although it's typically recommended to have a sponsor of the same gender, I was well into sobriety when I wasn't working with anyone. A friend asked, "If you could have any sponsor, who would it be?" and out blurted "Bill" from my mouth. I'd never thought to ask him, because I didn't want to "break the rules." But the more I entertained it, the more I knew working with a man was exactly what I needed. A man I already trusted and relied on.

When I asked Bill if he might sponsor me, I was frank about my tendency to sexualize relationships. We discussed how he was a mentor, slightly older and married, basically a recipe for disaster. Bill didn't seem phased. He knew he had strong boundaries and we decided to move forward. In all the years I have worked with him since, Bill and I have never had an ounce of difficulty. The old dynamic never came up.

When I talked with him about my reservations with Yancey, Bill said, "Ingrid, you have always tried to make the wrong person right, and now you are trying to make the right person wrong." He had a way of speaking directly to my sense of knowing, and it was a relief.

As I leaned into more of a relationship with Yancey, I experienced his healthy boundaries and honesty. He never tried to paint a rosy picture. In fact, Yancey said, "You seem great for me, but I understand if you don't feel the same." *He didn't gaslight me.* He honored my feelings of hesitation related to his drinking, he wasn't in a rush, he wanted me to feel safe.

We put all of our cards on the table from the get-go. I wanted a family, he thought it would be nice but wasn't attached to it. I am not an animal person and he had a cat. As we continued to deepen our relationship, we did the brave work of inviting reality into our discussions of building a life together. Neither one of us felt we had to compromise who we were as individuals in order to be together.

Yancey committed to sobriety when we committed to each other and it was the greatest relief. He was the first person I had ever been with who didn't drink. I never worried about coming home to him drunk, that he would drive drunk, or that his personality would change at dinner.

But I did continue pointing out everything else I thought he was doing "wrong." Drops of water on the floor after he showered or the way he didn't get under the sheets. I couldn't stop micromanaging. Not because I didn't trust him, but because I still had a nervous system that ran on high alert. Yancey seemed to accept this about me, and when I apologized for overstepping, he would easily forgive.

We always did what we said we were going to, rather than dreaming and dragging our feet. On our first date, we randomly talked about the flying trapeze and later found ourselves swinging upside down, overlooking the Santa Monica Pier. We felt like kids running off to the circus and if I do say so myself, we were some of the best students in class.

When you are pushing forty, and experience something so radically different and fulfilling, you don't need much of a test-drive. Before I could start obsessing and worrying, Yancey proposed to me in a way that actually caught me by surprise.

He bought me a beautiful ring, a generous gift, and I loved the symbol of our commitment, but I didn't need a symbol this time. We talked about getting married at my cousin's farm in Colorado, but my uncle had recently passed away and I knew my cousin Megan was in deep grief. I didn't want to put any pressure on her and wondered if we should even ask.

But before we got off the phone with Megan, she had created a Pinterest board for everything she wanted to do with her property. Our wedding gave her the motivation to do it, and in six short months, she turned her previously barren acres of land into a literal flower farm. Dahlias the size of dinner plates, zinnias in bright shades of fuchsia, coral and yellow. You would think Megan had been flower farming her whole life given the crops that awaited us in August of 2014.

It was the perfect backdrop for our dearest friends and family to come together, holding parasols in the bright Colorado sun, surrounding a burlap runner on the expansive green lawn. We had a bluegrass band, long tables for a family style Italian feast, outdoor chandeliers and vintage sofas brought out from Megan's antique barn. Pinterest had come to life.

The fact that Randy was in attendance was a major thorn for me, but like so many other occasions, I had to tolerate him if I were to be in relationship with my mom. I really wanted her at my wedding and I felt better equipped to deal with Randy's presence than I could bear to have her choose him over me again.

As a wedding gift, Randy contributed his sound system for the event and his large speakers were positioned outside the cottage house. It was threatening rain all day and there were huge gusts of wind. When Yancey tried to be helpful by moving the speakers under cover, Randy scolded him like a child. It was a mild moment in comparison to many others in my life, but enough for Yancey to get his own taste of my childhood.

Gatherings where both sides of my family got together were extremely rare, but there we were: two parents, two stepparents, four step brothers, two stepsisters and my biological brother Josh. And we all coexisted without major incident, almost. My stepmom, Alice, approached me immediately after the ceremony. "Your dad and I are really tired so we're going home."

"What? We haven't had dinner. We haven't had the father/daughter dance." I was surprised when I continued, "You are welcome to go. In fact, I will call you a cab, but you are *not* taking my dad with you." Imagine a really nasty tone coming from a truly beautiful bride.

Alice ended up staying and sulking off to the side for much of the night, but I tried to ignore her. My dad walked the fine line of saying, "She is my wife and I'm not going to talk bad about her," but he also said he wouldn't leave.

I danced with my dad at my wedding and I'm so glad I fought for that moment. He was smiling so big as he twirled me around like a professional dancer, wearing a charcoal gray suit and fedora. I will treasure the photographs of that experience the rest of my life.

Dancing with my dad and having him walk me down the aisle felt like we were the quintessential father/daughter duo. The fact that this happened right as he was descending into memory loss made me wish I could freeze time. No matter what else had happened, my dad was the man who wanted to rescue me as a child, and who would later come to whisk me away under a suspended chandelier and moonlight, looking at me with nothing but love.

Later in the evening, I surprised Yancey by singing *At Last* by Etta James. Truer lyrics were never sung. Then our friends and family started giving beautiful speeches. Because the microphone belonged to Randy, he imagined himself to be the emcee. Between each toast, he'd stand there in his bright orange t-shirt, the outfit he deemed fit for my wedding, reveling in the spotlight. It made me so angry.

Yancey held my hand under the table, trying to regulate my blood pressure, but even he almost choked when Randy grabbed the mic after my high school girlfriends spoke. He said, "Yay for high school friends!" and then in a more sinister tone, "I've always loved high school girls, hahaha."

I gritted my teeth. I wouldn't let him ruin this day. Twelve days shy of my fortieth birthday, I wasn't running and I wasn't looking to be saved. I stood before God, my family, and friends as I said marriage vows to a stable, present, and loving partner who was looking back at me: a stable, present, and loving partner.

Randy could have worn a bright orange jumpsuit. It made no difference if he were happy for us or gave me the silent treatment that day. Walking down the aisle, in the middle of my cousin's farm, I only had eyes for Yancey and we were surrounded by more tenderness than our hearts could hold. I felt at peace, and as though I'd finally arrived in the here and now. Perhaps I was finally moving out of constant survival. I could love and be loved.

24

What Does She Think
About *Me*?

Less than two years after that idyllic day, I would be
back in Colorado at my cousin's farm, hearing my
mom say that Randy had cancer. Nine months after
that, I was flying back with Henry to see her in the
wake of Randy's death.

My brother Josh picked us up in Denver, and the
three of us drove several hours towards Westcliffe,
Colorado: population 417. I had never heard of the
remote town before my mom and Randy moved there.
As Josh pulled up to the house, our mom came outside.
It was early January and about ten degrees, so she was
bundled in her huge parka. I got Henry out of his seat
and we all went inside.

As I hugged my mom, I noticed that the invisible
barrier we had always had was still there. And as I stood
in her house, it became clear that what had changed

in me immediately following Randy's death hadn't changed us. I wanted to feel like the thing that made me feel safer made her feel safer too, but it didn't.

My mom had tears in her eyes, but she was trying to shake them off. "I'm so glad you are here," she said. "Are you guys hungry?" People had brought casseroles and even a high chair for Henry. It was nice to focus on the simplicity of preparing food and watching Henry try ham for the first time. It was like we all bracketed out what had just happened, a lifetime of hurt before it, and were just leaning into being together.

But the longer we sat at the kitchen table, the more I looked around and saw Randy in every piece of furniture and art on the walls. In more ways than one, this was not the "new" situation I was hoping for. He was still so *present.*

I went a little numb. *I know how to do this. It's not about me. Focus on being helpful.* I decided that a "real" relationship with my mom might take more time.

The next morning, I found a bag of dried beans in my mom's cupboard and poured them into a large plastic bowl. I set it on the floor with some cups and spoons, hoping to occupy Henry while my mom and I pulled out her laptop. We needed to dive into her bank accounts and bills.

I could see my mom was anxious to show me her competence, as though she needed to prove to *me* she was capable. This was the first time she had ever lived alone. My mom went from her parents' house to marrying my dad to living with Randy. She wasn't sure if she could take care of all the things that needed managing.

Technology was intimidating for my mom. Largely because Randy used to be her only teacher and he went out of his way to make her feel stupid. You could hear the frustration and ridicule in his voice when he spoke to her. He also knew all of my mom's passwords and monitored everything, so she had no autonomy or privacy.

His own privacy however, was paramount. Randy was famous for convoluted and paranoid systems for the most mundane of tasks.

But despite his best efforts in life, Randy's secrets were starting to come to the surface. As my mom and I starting looking at her accounts, I was shocked to see how much credit card debt they had. Neither of them had really worked in years, and I thought it was because they had done so well selling their business and the ranch they bought after I left high school. Randy also received some inheritance when his parents passed away.

But it was becoming clear they were under water. And several of the credit cards were in my mom's name only. "What were those used for?" I asked.

"Well, I recently found out that Randy had a secret P.O. box in Austin, Texas," she said.

"What are you talking about?" My tone was bitter. I couldn't help myself.

"I guess he opened up a mailbox down there so I wouldn't know about it. He had several credit card statements going there and some of them were in my name. I didn't even know they existed."

"This is fraud, Mom! You shouldn't have to pay those cards!" This was another level to his longstanding financial abuse. Randy made it difficult for my mom to earn her own money and kept her in the dark about everything else. I was furious and trying to tap into her rage, but she didn't seem to have any.

"I just want to pay it and be done," she said.

"But you didn't take out those cards! You shouldn't be responsible for them!"

"I know I didn't, but I can't prove that. This is too stressful and I have too much to do already with having to pack up and sell this house. I can't deal with anything else. I closed the P.O. box and I don't even want to know what else was going there."

I wanted to know what else was going there. I wanted to know all of his secrets. They were a strange comfort to me. But I understood where my mom was coming from. She had to sell the house they once owned or the bank was going to take it back. Years earlier, Randy had taken out a reverse mortgage. My mom just lost her husband and now she had to pack up a life and find a new one, all without his help.

Henry dumped the black beans all over the floor and was starting to get fussy. I scooped up the mess and tried rocking him in the living room while my mom finished up on her computer.

I was feeling rather small, sitting in Randy's house, rocking my son to sleep. For the first time in years, I was looking at all of his *things*. My childhood was everywhere and I felt assaulted.

The triggers were starting to pile up, and I felt less stable with each passing day. My body became stiff, my headaches got worse. It's like I was swelling up underneath an iron wardrobe and the pressure was building.

My mom seemed more stable than I was anticipating—she had even stayed away from any wine, and I was grateful. But several days into my visit, the bottle came out of hiding.

Henry was asleep and we were watching TV in the living room. Chatting about nothing, her words were getting sloppy. Her mood was shifting. She was suddenly bitter and bringing up all kinds of things we had never talked about before.

I felt like she was channeling Randy. Her voice sounded like his, the words she used were straight from his mouth. She started talking about Randy's eldest daughter and son, Stacy and Sean, saying things I'd heard Randy say before.

"Stacy is bipolar and crazy, and Sean is only out for himself. Every time we tried to help him, he fucked it up." She sounded *exactly* like Randy, confident and entitled. It was as if Randy had written a script for my mom to keep repeating after he'd gone. I saw that his lies had become her truth.

Not only were these things make-believe, they were void of any role Randy had in his relationships with his kids. It was painful to hear. I tried to rationalize with her. "Mom, I'm a psychologist, I think I would know if Stacy had bipolar disorder! This whole conversation feels ridiculous." No matter what I said, she didn't hear me. She got louder in her opinions and I wasn't going to change her mind.

My own sanity and connection to my mom had hung on the notion that she was still *in there*. That she would never believe such malicious fantasies about people she personally knew and loved. But here she was, telling me these things as though they were facts, even after Randy was gone. I felt horrible for Stacy and Sean, and humiliated for myself. All these years, I had given her the benefit of the doubt.

I told her I didn't want to talk about it anymore and I was going to bed. Henry was in the crib in our room and I really wanted to call Yancey, so I couldn't go in there. I couldn't go outside because it was freezing, so I went to the only place in the house I could have some privacy, Randy's office.

My phone was about to die, so I started searching for a plug. There was a power strip under Randy's desk so I sat on the floor, tied to the three-foot leash.

"Oh my God, what was I thinking?" I said to Yancey. "I can't believe I'm here. That I disrupted my life, completely disrupted Henry's life, taking him to the freezing cold and a house that reeks of abuse to take care of someone who never took care of me. Who never believed me and probably never will. I feel like such a fool."

I was crying hard, yet trying to stay quiet so my mom couldn't hear from her bedroom upstairs. I told Yancey about the conversation we'd just had about Stacy and Sean. "What does she think about me? What the fuck does she still think about *me*?"

I was in a heap on the office floor. Any self-respect I had garnered by my willingness to postpone the trip until after Randy died had drained from my body. I was flattened and didn't know what to do. Yancey mostly listened as I freaked out for over an hour.

"And I can't believe I'm calling you from *Randy's office*. It's like he's still here. I'm sitting next to his filing cabinets—probably full of more secrets my mom doesn't know about. It's like even his photos are staring back at me in disgust."

I was starting to feel a little lighter, the more I talked. Yancey supported me no matter what I needed to do, even if that meant coming home early. I was certainly thinking about it. I was exhausted, completely tapped out. At some point, I knew I just needed sleep.

"I love you so much," Yancey said. "You're going to be okay no matter what."

"Okay. I love you too. I'll call you in the morning." I hung up, got off the floor, and tiptoed into the guest bedroom next door. Looking down at Henry in the dark room, I found his breath calming. Like I could regulate my own breathing by matching it with his. I wanted to pick him up to snuggle, but I didn't dare wake him.

I got under the covers and drifted off quickly. I woke up to Henry's noises and scooped him out of the crib. We both went into the living room and my mom was already up and seemed cheerful. I was surprised how different things felt. Like the proverbial "new day," it was hard to access the part of me who was seriously thinking about leaving the night before.

I wondered if my mom even remembered our conversation. We never spoke of it again. In our typical fashion, the dysfunction was set aside and we went back to the other part of our relationship. The one where we didn't address the elephants in the room and we got along.

We also never spoke about my decision to postpone our trip until after Randy passed away. Why would we talk about any of these things when we hadn't discussed my relationship with him since our therapy session in the early 90s? My not running to his deathbed was the first time I had "confronted" our past at all since it happened.

But in our silence, I had always interpreted a collective "knowing." Now I wondered if I had been endowing my mom with more awareness than she ever had. I had always believed her ability to overlook my pain was because she was overlooking her own. I had given her a pass. But things were changing. I hoped her new life might give her the freedom to re-inhabit her old self, a version that wouldn't deny her daughter's reality. But that didn't seem to be happening.

***

Not long after I returned home, my mom left a message saying she'd had a really hard weekend. I didn't get a chance to call her back right away but when I did, I wanted to encourage her to talk about her grief. I thought it was a good sign she was feeling her feelings.

When she answered, my mom began crying. I could tell within seconds that she'd been drinking. Surprisingly, it didn't bother me too much. She was still coherent and we were able to carry on a conversation.

But then she switched from talking about her sadness to talking about Josh. He was coming back to see her that weekend. "I honestly don't know what I would do without him. I'm just so proud of everything he's done and how he's turned his life around." She was so effusive about how much she loved him and how amazed she was about his sobriety. She went on for a good five minutes about how incredibly meaningful their relationship was.

I was getting more and more irritated. I had been sober for half of my life. I had always privileged my mom's security over my own, but she still only had eyes for her baby boy. I had to purse my lips to keep from blurting out: "I know, Mom, Josh is your beloved and favorite child."

I knew my mom's love and gratitude was warranted. There was a period of decades I thought we had lost my brother to his addiction. His sweet and tender heart had become obscured by anger and he said the most hateful things when he was drunk, all of which I blocked from my memory. He vacillated between jail and homelessness until, shortly after Randy got sick, Josh checked himself in to the Salvation Army. Right when I thought he would never get sober, he did.

The way Josh turned his life around *was* worthy of praise. Over the last year, he had been there for our mom in ways I could never be. But listening to her on the phone, I could practically see her beaming with pride. And I had never heard her talk about me the way she talked about Josh. Not about my sobriety, education, career, or my family. The disparity was agonizing.

As though she finally had a moment of self-awareness, or perhaps noticed my silence, my mom's tone changed to one of awkwardness, maybe even a little embarrassed. "And you know, I love you too," she said.

I took a deep breath and closed my eyes. "Yes, Mom, I know. I love you too. I actually have to get going for preschool pickup."

I wanted to throw my phone and scream. I couldn't keep pretending my mom didn't tell us both that Josh was her favorite child. I couldn't keep tolerating how she saw me as a spiteful girl who made her life miserable. And I knew more than her children, Randy was always her favorite. He won the favor of her protection.

I wanted my mom in my life. I wanted Henry to know his grandmother. But I was becoming aware of how much I had given up already, how much of myself I had been sacrificing all these years. Now that Randy was gone, I didn't want to do it anymore. I didn't think I could.

25

I Am Here

Not long after that phone call with my mom, I was in my therapist's office. I couldn't express anger out in the world, but I was starting to access it with Kristi in a way that felt safe. Prior to these recent sessions, I had grown to hate the process of therapy. I was *over* my own story, the one that remained the same no matter how far I got from it.

But something about this work felt different. I'd started a clinical training in Somatic Experiencing (SE), a trauma therapy, not because I thought I had PTSD but because I wanted to help my clients with nervous system regulation. As a part of the training, we had to work with a somatic experiencing practitioner ourselves.

Kristi had sort of a hippie vibe, with flowy clothing and wavy hair. She sat cross-legged in her arm chair, which I loved and judged at the same time. I think we were close in age, but I always felt like people my own age were so much older. Maybe I wanted to see her as a mother figure, so age didn't really matter.

I was telling her the story about how much my mom loved my brother when I suddenly felt a feeling I identified as rage. "I feel *so angry!*" I said, and then quickly returned to the content of the phone call.

"I'm wondering if you would be willing to return to the feeling for a moment?" Kristi asked. She looked comfortable and kind, and I hated her for just a second. *Ugh, I don't want to return to the feeeeling, just let me tell you what happened and then we can move on!*

Sitting across from her, I tried to set aside my disgust (and the thought I had done something wrong by fleeing the feeling in the first place). I closed my eyes and started to become curious about what was happening in my body: the heat that was on my shoulders and the fire in my belly. "This is so fucking annoying!" I said with as much volume as I allowed myself in her office.

I opened my eyes and looked around. I caught a glimpse of a coaster that was sitting on her side table. I'd never seen it before. It was a made of adobe, imprinted with the red rays of the New Mexico state flag. Randy was from Albuquerque and we had the same set of coasters in my house growing up. It was strange seeing an artifact that represented my childhood sitting in my therapist's office.

The visual seemed to amplify what was brewing, unbelievable anger over a lifelong pursuit of external validation that never came. "If I couldn't get it from my parents, then I was going to find it *somewhere* … maybe in achievement after achievement," I said. "I've run a marathon, received three college degrees, published a book, and none of these have been a teeny tiny drop in the bucket of the healing I was longing to get from them."

Kristi nodded. I felt like a cliché but also found her presence immensely helpful. *Ugh. I hate this!*

"I'm not saying these things weren't worthy of my time and I'm proud of what I've done, but the part of me that was doing these things to *overcome* is pissed it hasn't worked!"

The rage that welled up inside me was a rare glimpse of what I knew was always there, conscious-adjacent. As I allowed myself to feel even a fraction of it, an image of thrusting my fist directly in front of me appeared.

The fantasy of my balled-up hand throwing a punch replayed over and over in slow-motion. I saw my fist intersect with a metal wall, the impact shattering the wall into millions of pieces a foot away from my face. I was narrating all of this to Kristi as though it were a movie she couldn't see. "I can see the pieces starting to fly in every direction," I said.

"Keep going. Notice what you're experiencing as you feel that punch and see the wall shatter."

I heard her ask me to stay with my experience, with my body, but I immediately went back into my head and thought *This seems typical.* I analyzed the fantasy as a representation of what I was sure would happen if I actually felt my anger: it would come back to hurt me.

Except, when I finally returned to what my body was telling me, it didn't feel afraid. My body didn't want me to stop. I needed to keep going. This felt important.

Kristi trusted my process and asked, "Is there anything that can protect you from the shards of metal?"

I immediately saw myself covered in ancient armor. I checked in with my body to see if the image felt sufficient. Once I was safe behind the mail that covered my face and metal breastplate that secured my torso, I saw the shards flying at me faster and harder, almost like I was a magnet. I was no longer punching the fictitious wall, but pieces were originating out of thin air, like a summer rain was coming down hard and horizontal.

The fragments were coming directly for me, and the harder they landed, the greater the sound of metal on metal. I could hear it in my mind and feel it reverberating throughout my body. It was visceral, exhilarating, the pounding and vibrating like a tribal dance on my chest. The vibration was such that I started to spontaneously say, "I am here, I am here, I am here."

There was no mistaking what was being revealed. *My whole self is here.* All the ways I sought to feel present and worthy up until that moment had never brought me to this place. It was allowing the millions of shards of shrapnel that would certainly come for me if ever I were to stop and be me that allowed me to feel whole, here, and alive.

Not only could I handle the sharp edges that were gunning for me, I wanted more because they felt so *good*. I needed to multiply them in my mind, to give myself the full impact. Louder, harder, hitting every inch of my body. It wasn't a punishment. It was an awakening. My rage gave that to me.

The energy started to pour through me in a circular motion. It started at my back, a current that ran like a river through my heart and out again. It was coming from behind, not out in front of me like a milestone I needed to achieve. It was ushering me forward and coming through me without my management.

I felt compelled to intensify the energy and asked Kristi if I could throw the small beanbag I'd been holding. It was the same size as my phone. She said it was fine, so I surprisingly let the pillow fly across the room with as much force as I could put behind it.

Then the tears came. I closed my eyes and started sobbing. I was blown away by how mysteriously I was being guided to the healing. I couldn't have dreamt that such a powerful moment would arise, and that it had something to do with images of violent punches and sharp metal. I didn't need to come up with a treatment plan for myself. I needed to get out of my own way, to let the feelings come, to trust the truth in my body so I could begin to reclaim it. And it was witnessed by someone who could help me integrate this wisdom even further. Another layer of healing. Another layer of grief, sloughed away. Essential pieces of me uncovered, making me more whole.

Part Three: Trauma Healing

"As traumatized children we always dreamed that someone would come and save us. We never dreamed that it would, in fact, be ourselves, as adults."

— Alice Little

26

Me Too

Ever since I'd been to my mom's after Randy died, it felt like the eraser of a pencil was being driven into the side of my bicep. I tried everything to alleviate the pain: massage, arnica, Advil, but nothing worked. After six months I couldn't raise my arm above ninety degrees. I had to put on my bra like a thirteen-year-old, fastening it in front before swinging it around back. An MRI revealed I had "frozen shoulder," so I became the lucky recipient of twice-weekly physical therapy.

It was a typical sunny day in Los Angeles as I drove away from Henry's preschool. Heading north towards Larchmont Boulevard, I was listening to NPR when I heard a reference to Harvey Weinstein. I'd been following that story somewhat closely and became curious about a tape that had surfaced.

They weren't going to play it, so I pulled over to see if I could find it on my iPhone, wanting to hear what was so scandalous. I quickly found a link, pressed play, and merged back into traffic.

A woman had secretly recorded Harvey berating her as she tried to protect herself from his abuse of power. Listening to the recording, I saw the color draining from my knuckles as I clutched the steering wheel. *I know that voice.* My body became as still as it could while still operating a vehicle. I was being transported back in time as I listened to the familiar tone of disgust and manipulation.

I knew I was having a personal "me too" moment, but it extended beyond the sexual abuse I was hearing in surrounding reports. It was the tone in Harvey's voice: his contempt, lack of empathy or remorse. It was his narcissism. *It was Randy.*

I was suddenly a little girl driving a big car, and grateful the recording was over in one and a half minutes. I turned off my phone and turned on the radio. I tried connecting to the present moment through my senses—consciously feeling the seat beneath me, allowing it to support me more fully. I changed the radio station to some music I could sing to. I needed to change the energy of that moment, fleeing it as fast as I could.

I started piecing something together I hadn't really known before, something else that had been missing in all my personal therapy. Whether my therapists were men or women, seasoned or newly trained, not once did any of them mention the words, "gaslighting," "psychological abuse," "grooming," or "narcissism." Words I was hearing related to Harvey Weinstein. No one put my story into this context. I didn't know how narcissism presented as a kid, and then no one ever mentioned Randy might fit that bill.

This, this is what I experienced.

I had learned about narcissism in graduate school, but it was an academic presentation, not related to the man who walked around my house in his underwear when I was a child. Connections were being made in my brain that had never linked up.

As I got closer to the medical building on Larchmont, I was grateful to find a parking spot and feel my feet on the ground. I met with my physical therapist and knew she was the perfect person to see that morning. Her ability to bring me back into my body with gentle touch was just what I needed.

She worked on me for an hour and I left feeling more in my body, with a tad more flexibility. I got back in my car and headed towards my office, driving in silence, and began to notice several lines emerging in my mind, almost like a poem.

I had never written this way, in this style or voice. More lines followed and I felt driven to capture them exactly as they had appeared. I had a feeling they would be gone as quickly as they came. I grabbed my phone and began to dictate. With one hand on the steering wheel, the other holding my phone, I said out loud to myself in the car:

I didn't exist unless I was serving a fantasy or function
for him.
In my early teens, he secretly professed his love to me.
Telling me how haunted he was about his feelings.
I told him I was glad he was talking about it.
But I probably wasn't the appropriate person to tell.
This made him angry.
And once again, I was a ghost.

When he felt smitten, he showered me with attention
and gifts.
Inappropriate gifts.
Jewelry that was too expensive.
Club memberships we couldn't afford.
When he felt guilty, he was too ashamed to look at
me.
And the smallest infraction would invite steep
punishment.

He stole my journals.
Quoted me back to me.
Claiming omniscience.
Ripping my vulnerability to shreds.

When he came back to my room one night.
I saw the vacancy in his eyes.
As he went in to kiss me.
And then kiss me again.

I yelled his name as I pushed him off of me in the
doorway.
He visibly came back into his body.
And turned to walk away.

He would time my showers.
Five minutes or less.
Standing just outside the door.
Where my naked body bathed.
Did he do this to his son?
I don't seem to recall.

He pulled me out of school and took me to Las
Vegas.
Las Vegas.
Without my mother's consent.
Behind her back.
While she was with her dying father in Texas.

He lied to my brothers and said we were all staying
with friends that weekend.
He was going "out of town on business."
He told me to lie to my brothers and to say the same.
He told me to pack my bag, but to leave it hidden.
We would get it later when no one was looking.

He told me on the plane I could never tell anyone.
He told me on the plane he only got one hotel room.
This trip was costing him a fortune already.

He took me on a shopping spree.
Told me I had to dress older.
Said I had to hold his hand to look older so they
wouldn't kick me out.

In about ten minutes, the lines stopped coming and the composition felt complete. I'd never talked about these experiences so succinctly, like bullet point facts.

I pulled up to a stoplight on La Brea and noticed the gas station on the corner. The large Chevron sign had always been there, but the reds and blues were suddenly vibrant. It felt like a veil had been lifted from my eyes, I was seeing things so clearly. I suddenly felt connected with my surroundings, like I wasn't alone in my car anymore. People on the street corner, sitting in the cars next to me, it was as though I'd just dropped into my body, no longer on autopilot and moving through the world ... but actually *in* it.

I arrived at my office fifteen minutes later and read what I had written. It felt important and I kept reviewing the lines, the truth of them penetrating. It was as though naming what happened in such a clear and concise way was closing a gap between what I had always known, and how I later came to see it. Like I was attempting to return to the unfiltered truth without minimizing.

The poem was a stand-alone piece for about a week. I wanted to share it, but wasn't sure how or when. Then I started seeing #metoo posts on Facebook. It seemed I wasn't alone in wanting to break my silence, naming what I had been through. I decided to share my piece, grateful my mom wasn't on social media at the time and I could be "public" without upsetting her.

It felt empowering to have a voice in this way. But I felt like I needed *more*. The experience didn't feel complete. Several days later, essays started coming as abruptly and forcefully as the poem. Beginning from the outer edges of my personal experiences, they started to circle around my pain, moving closer and closer to the heart of it. My first marriage and divorce, my alcoholism and sobriety, all the ways I didn't trust or know myself.

I didn't think I could write the whole "Randy story." I truly didn't want to. The lines in the poem were as deep as I wanted to go. But eventually it felt as though I had no choice. All of these essays were winding their way back to him. And when I gave myself permission to capture *everything*, I started writing thirty pages a day.

In between clients and taking care of Henry, I felt a sense of profound urgency as I dictated into my phone story after story. While my literal defenses were down, between my waking and dream life, usually at 3:00 a.m., my eyes would pop open and I would have to get out of bed, tiptoe to my kitchen table and open my computer. It almost felt manic, and I would have been concerned if I didn't recognize this as the voice I had been sitting on for thirty years.

213

I had kept my experiences compartmentalized for so long, it was like huge parts of me were totally walled off. As I started writing, with some notion of sharing it, my body felt like I had already shouted from the rooftops: "This is my *truth*!" and it felt incredible. With each and every sentence, I was reclaiming myself.

I shared my writing at the end of each day with Yancey. "You wrote all of this *today*?" he asked. He was stunned by what was pouring out of me, and how coherent it was. It was like these fully formed essays had just been waiting for me to be ready.

"This is the most helpful and healing thing I've ever done for myself," I told him. "And I just can't stop."

For the first time in my life, I wasn't compulsively pursuing healing—healing was pursuing me. I felt a calling to go within, to the depths, to restore what had always been there. I'd grown so tired of looking for *something* or *someone* to lift me higher or to prove my worth. Tired of chasing relief. No longer censored out of fear, I was giving myself a voice.

My writing emerged from a place of obscurity, trying to crawl out from under something I still couldn't put my finger on. But by wading into what felt like mysterious and murky waters, I was giving language and context to experiences that were previously hidden. I understood why I never could have healed prior to my writing because I couldn't name what I was healing *from*. Now, with every word

I wrote, I was owning my story. Saying to my younger self: *I believe you and we will finally find a way through.*

27

Pain Porn

I didn't set out to write a memoir. I certainly didn't want to write a book about childhood trauma from narcissistic abuse. *I didn't even know that's what I was writing.* I just felt compelled to capture these stories. I needed to admit all the ways I'd struggled and coped. There was something I was piecing together, like a giant puzzle of my life.

But before I could sort it out and see the big picture, the process itself was becoming more difficult. The subject matter was, in fact, terrifying. This was nothing like writing a dissertation or academic book. It was so personal! And I'd never written anything like it, so I didn't know how.

I asked for a lot of help, but critiques on my writing felt like pushback on my story. The triggers were unbearable and many times I tried convincing Yancey I was making a huge mistake.

"I'm trying to write about not being seen and how painful that was, and I have to write it in a way that makes people care. No one cared back then. Why would they care now? It's like I'm throwing myself in the fire one more time!"

Yancey listened and tried to encourage me, but I didn't want to hear it.

I eventually took my pain and confusion to Kristi's office. "Fuck all this uncovering, the memories I've buried or never looked at closely. Why would I want to fine tune them one sentence at a time?" I was ranting. "Is this going to help me somehow? As usual, I've been thinking how it might help others, but is it going to help me?"

Kristi gave me a look that seemed to say, *keep going.*

"I want to run from the shit that doesn't feel good. After all this time, I can still barely tolerate these feelings. I just look for the next thing and the next thing that might fix them until there is no more next. Just the ground, just the weight of it, maybe even burying me alive."

Perhaps I was being a bit dramatic, but I couldn't stop.

"All this writing feels like pain porn. How can I swing so far from one end of the spectrum, where I felt like I was putting the pieces together in a way that was so gratifying, creative and self-honoring… It does *not* feel that way today."

I took up the entire session venting. When I was finally ready to hear Kristi's thoughts, time was up. It's like that sometimes. So, I got back in my car and noticed I was still processing.

I knew there was something on the other side of this and I just had to get there. I suspected if I could finally acknowledge the big things that happened, the little things wouldn't feel so impossible. Maybe I could let Yancey hug me without feeling like it forced me to feel everything I'd stuffed down.

So, I kept writing but I still judged myself for the timing. Like, *Why now?* I could answer with *Because it's the truth.* But the truth felt *mean.* Like I was trampling on my mom right after she lost her husband, and it was evidence for the spoiled brat they said I was.

All my second-guessing didn't really matter, because the rage inside kept building. No matter how much I tried to focus on "my side of the street," on forgiveness or moving on, it never saved me from the embers that were constantly radiating heat.

So, I kept going and the more I wrote, the more questions I had. I wondered if Randy had secret lives we never knew about? Arrest records? Dating profiles? I did several deep dives on the internet but didn't find anything incriminating.

Then I started asking questions about the life I did know. There were so many gaps in my memory, I realized I needed help constructing this puzzle. I felt compelled to find more "evidence." Like I needed to find every shred of truth that ever existed so I could finally possess my own.

I started by calling social services in Aspen, asking if they had any records from 1991. I wanted to see how the social workers viewed my situation. What were their actual recommendations? I wanted to see that meeting through their eyes, and through my own as a clinician now.

They saw that my family was in their system, but the old records were nowhere to be found. I continued my search, wondering if I could track down Karen, my school counselor or Cindy, our family therapist. I couldn't believe how bold I'd become, shamelessly searching for anyone that crossed my mind. When those roads went cold, I started turning towards my immediate circle.

Next to my mom, I knew John could be hurt the most by what I was writing. He was so close with his dad and I needed to talk with him about what was being stirred up. I also hoped to ask him some questions. I suspected there were things about Randy only he would know.

We hadn't been in regular touch over the years, but we reconnected a bit since his dad died, so I gave him a call. "Hi, John, I wanted to talk with you about something ... I am actually writing another book."

"I knew you were going to say that!" John replied.

I was blown away at his intuition. "Really? That's amazing! How did you know?"

"I read your Facebook post, the one with the poem. That was huge and I'm so glad you shared it. But I kind of suspected that more was going to come."

I was so relieved. It felt like he was already giving me some of the permission I was seeking. "Well, I know you and I had a very different relationship with your dad, and I don't want to hurt you in any way. This is just something I suddenly feel called to do. It's like I finally need to tell my side of the story."

"No, I totally get that," John said.

He was one hundred percent supportive, so I began asking questions about when we lived together, and about his time in Florida. John laughed when I reminded him about the mysterious caller asking for Ben Webber. "Yeah, I think the guy who gave my dad the Ben Webber ID was in a motorcycle gang. Ben Webber was his brother or something."

John went on to say he remembered living in a trailer Randy had rented from a family who lived on the same property when they got to Florida. On the Fourth of July, they were celebrating with their landlords and like many other nights, John fell asleep in one of the kid's rooms inside the house.

The next morning, all three kids woke up to the sound of more fireworks, *Boom, Boom, Boom!* Excited, they raced outside. The sound was coming from the trailer, so they went over to investigate. When they opened the door, they saw Randy sitting on the couch next to the other kids' mom. She was visibly shaking and crying. Standing above her was the kids' dad, pointing a gun at Randy.

"What?" I blurted. "This is such a crazy story."

"Yeah. They immediately tried to downplay it, saying the gunshots were blanks and no one was hurt. But a few years ago, my dad and I talked about that day and he told me they were live bullets and the guy just missed him."

John told me that living in Florida was a twenty-four-hour party. There was a lot of drinking, just like our childhood together, but with a lot more people coming and going. He was in little league and Randy was his coach; they always went to the beach. "It was a lot of fun," he said.

John *enjoyed* this time with his dad. Even now, he didn't seem mad that he was taken from his mom.

"I remember hearing your mom had detectives looking for you," I said, "that she had to pack up the house you'd been living in, boxing up your things, not knowing if she would ever see you again? All of that seemed so brutal to me."

"That is definitely the fucked-up part," John said. "We just never talked about my mom. It was like she wasn't in my life anymore, not in a bad way, just like a fact. It wasn't until I got older that I even became aware of how much that impacted my relationship with her."

John was gone for two and a half years. The idea that someone might take Henry from me ... it was too excruciating to contemplate.

I asked how it all ended and John said one day Randy called his mom, Teri. He told her where they were and that they were coming back to Colorado. "My mom had instructions to call the police if she ever heard from him, but she didn't want to hurt me in any way. So, she agreed to meet us by herself," he said. "I remember sort of *meeting* my mom for the first time that day. I was seven and my dad pointed out a woman with curly blonde hair standing across the room. She was a stranger to me."

Hearing these details completely broke my heart. John said it took at least ten years for him and his mom to be in "real relationship," and as we talked more about Teri, he told me she was only sixteen when she married Randy.

Sixteen.

"That's how old I was when he took me to Vegas," I said. This detail felt profound. *I was the same age as Teri.*

"And Angie was only seventeen when she lived with us in Florida," John said. "She was my dad's girlfriend for a long time."

Randy was in his thirties by that point. *Oh my God, this was a pattern!*

"Do you think your mom would be open to talking to me?" I asked without really thinking. "I wonder if there are other parallels to our experiences?"

"I can definitely ask her," John said.

"Okay, that would be amazing. It makes me nervous to imagine, but I think it could be helpful," I said.

John and I continued to talk, and while I kept asking questions about Randy, he kept coming back to my mom. "How can any parent in their right mind, if they were told their daughter was receiving sexual advances from their husband…" He couldn't wrap his head around it. "Why wouldn't they get the fuck out of there and press charges?"

I knew he was right. But I didn't have the same feelings about it as John. Even in this conversation, I felt like I had to protect my mom. To help John understand what it was like to be under the spell of a narcissist like Randy, and it removed any feelings I had about my mom's part in my story at all.

But in that moment, I caught a glimpse of *my* pattern, the spell that I was under. I could see the divide between what I knew intellectually and how I always responded, *Don't talk badly about my mom.* I was still trying to save her so she might save me back. Still abandoning myself, even as I was working so hard to reclaim my truth.

28

Tracing Paper

After John and I spoke, I felt more confident to reach out to Randy's other kids, Stacy and Sean. They each had their own complicated relationship with their dad and were incredibly supportive of me and my writing. It was a relief knowing I had permission from all of Randy's kids to share my story. None of them ever questioned my experience.

I still had no intention of talking to my mom. I just wasn't ready. I kept thinking I would talk to her after the book was written, and only if it was going to be published. Then I'd be "forced" to talk to her. Until then, it was my secret.

Then one day, I got a text from John. "My mom wants to talk with you about everything. She knows you'll be calling. Here's her number ..."

It was one thing to speak to my siblings, or to people who were a part of my experiences directly. Calling Teri felt different. I didn't have a relationship with her as much as she and I each had our own relationship with Randy. But I felt like this was going to be an important conversation, so I put my headphones in and opened my computer.

"Hello," she answered in the same bubbly voice I remembered.

We exchanged a few pleasantries and then she shocked me with her first sentence about Randy. "I was a victim of his too," she said. "I was only fifteen."

A victim?— I thought she saw their story as "young love"— and *too?* As in, she saw me as a victim? It was almost too much to take in. I started typing as fast as I could, concentrating on the details Teri was sharing. It was as though she was coloring in my own experiences with sharp details; the specific elements of her story were like tracing paper over my past.

She went back to the beginning when Randy lived with his first wife, Linda, just a few houses down from his parents. "Randy's mom was a schoolteacher," Teri said.

As she brought up Dolores, I remembered the stories Randy told me about his mom, saying she was cruel and controlling. We had visited Albuquerque once or twice when I was in middle school.

Dolores had bright, Crayola red hair and perfume that got stuck in my nose. I instantly remembered she was a terrible cook. She made huge quantities of food for every meal and it all tasted the same, with a rancid overtone. I couldn't eat it, but it was clear we were not to disrespect Dolores.

One day, I spilled some juice in her kitchen. She came in and found me with a wad of paper towels in my hands. "You shouldn't take things without asking!" she scowled as though I were stealing.

Teri's recollection of Dolores continued and it brought me out of my reverie. She told me Dolores had an affair and that Randy went on secret outings with his mom to meet her "friend" when he was young, not knowing he was actually seeing his biological father. I realized how many lies Randy had grown up with too. How he'd been living in his own ill-fitting puzzle.

Teri said she knew Randy through her older brother, John. "They were best friends and Randy was always coming around our house," she said. "Big John" was eight years older than Teri and she was fifteen when he left Albuquerque. "Even after John was gone, Randy kept coming by."

One day, Randy called Teri and asked if she'd like to babysit, saying he'd make it "worth her while." She didn't really know Randy's kids, and was surprised by the job offer, but asked her parents if it was okay. Randy picked her up that Saturday night and they were about to drive away when he turned to her with a mischievous grin, saying, "I knew you just needed to get of that house. My mom is watching the kids tonight while you and I go to a basketball game."

"He literally tricked you into going to a basketball game?" My stomach was churning.

"I couldn't understand why he'd made up such a lie," Teri continued, "or why he wanted to take me. But he was right, I wanted to get out of the house. I'd already tried running away three times. My brother John probably told him all of that. And I wanted the attention. So, I went with it."

When the game was over, Randy invited her to his house, saying that Linda was working late. When they got there, he put on a record and made them both a Tom Collins—her first drink, ever—and sat next to her on the couch. "I sort of froze and then he kissed me," she said.

I immediately saw the moment where Randy kissed me in my bedroom doorway, how his eyes were vacant when he leaned towards my face.

Teri continued telling me how Randy had taken her home that night, and then kept calling, telling her how beautiful she was. She felt irresistible and started sneaking out to see Randy almost every night.

"He was still married, but said he wanted to marry me. Linda finally asked for a divorce and then I never received an official proposal. He just showed up one day with a pear-shaped diamond he'd bought from Zales where he worked."

A pear-shaped ring, for no particular reason. Hers was a diamond, but still …

"I accepted it but told him I didn't want to get married until I graduated from high school and turned eighteen."

I was clenching my stomach as Teri kept talking, bracing myself.

"Then, five days after my sixteenth birthday, Randy picked me up for school like usual, but I quickly realized we were heading in the wrong direction." She paused. "He took me to Mexico to get married."

I felt like thin arrows were shooting me from every angle, going straight through my body. I sat still, not moving an inch. If we hadn't been on the phone, or if I could have slowed time, I would have started bawling. The kind of cry that brings you to your knees. *Randy said he was taking her to school and then he didn't. He tricked her into getting married.*

They drove four hours to Juarez where Randy spoke with several men in Spanish, handing them cash. Their ceremony was in a nondescript office where Teri was wearing the clothes she'd worn to school that day. They stayed in a beautiful hotel that night and in the morning went straight to her parents' house.

"Didn't they try and contest the marriage or get you out of it somehow?" I asked.

"No," Teri said. "I actually think my dad was relieved to be rid of me. So, I just went to my bedroom and packed a small suitcase. I even grabbed my huge teddy bear, and then Randy and I left the house."

"I need to catch my breath a minute here," I said.

Teri was so young she'd grabbed *a teddy bear.* These particulars felt so important. They validated my own story more than anything ever had. I believed every word she told me. Randy was the liar. He was the manipulator. My own reality had been refuted for so long, even by my own mom, it erased some of my clarity and confidence. But listening to Teri was breathing life into my atrophied truth, giving it shape and color. It was exhilarating.

It was also terrifying. The resurrected pulse of my memory made my story more real than it had ever felt. Like I was really feeling the truth of it for the first time. A deep sadness welled up. Being assaulted by such a powerful feeling made me question, *Why am I doing this to myself?*

I had always talked with my clients as though this was the holy grail of mental health: integration, owning *all* the parts of ourselves—but in this moment, being a whole person made me want to vomit.

A part of me wanted to get off the phone, to stop the conversation, but I couldn't walk away. I sat glued to the chair at my kitchen table feeling like a slug: A large and sticky slug looking for anything to give me skin, to hold me in, to keep it all together knowing this is what I'd called for—the truth.

"Okay, I'm ready to go on," I said, just gritting my teeth.

I listened in a half-fog as Teri told me how she finished her junior and senior years with a husband, stepchildren, in-laws and her husband's ex-wife. She remembered Linda was always seeking child support, but Randy tried to get out of it. "He kept his finances a secret. As Stacy and Sean got older, Randy even told them to lie to their mom when they noticed an upgrade in our lifestyle so he wouldn't have to give more money."

He started blaming Teri for losing his family, saying he gave up his kids just to be with her. "I'll never forget the first time he got violent with me. He grabbed me by the hair and slammed my head against the car." Her life went on that like for two years before Teri turned eighteen and graduated high school. They moved to Colorado, where she hoped things might change.

Months later she found out she was pregnant, and was twenty-one when she had John. Though she loved him with all her heart, she could no longer stand the sight of Randy. One night she heard him come home around 2:00 a.m. "How come you're so cold to me?" he yelled with booze on his breath, shaking her by the shoulders. Before she could answer, Randy picked Teri up and threw her out the front door.

"I'll go, but not without my son!" She ran to the back door of the house and grabbed John from his crib, racing to her car. As they were about to drive off, she saw Randy standing there, yanking on the door. "He was in his underwear, screaming at me, trying to get in the car as we backed out the driveway."

She found a new place for her and John, but Randy kept stalking, parking near the house, going through her mail, so she got a restraining order. When the police knocked on Randy's door, he answered with a gun in his hand. He was taken to the hospital, admitted for suicidal ideation and a seventy-two-hour hold.

He was eventually served the restraining order in the hospital and Teri immediately pursued a divorce. What she didn't know at the time was that Randy had opened a secret P.O. box in Denver.

Another secret P.O. box.

It's where he had their $6,000 tax refund sent. When the check arrived, he forged Teri's name and cashed it. Then he picked up John from preschool on a Friday and Teri thought she'd have him back on Sunday as usual, but they never showed. She pleaded with the police for help, but the district attorney told her it wasn't really kidnapping if a boy was with his father.

I sat almost lifeless on the other end of the phone. We had talked for so long I was about to miss my doctor's appointment, and yet there was so much more to say. Before we said goodbye, I asked Teri how she was able to recover from everything she went through. After reflecting on the memories she'd just shared, the ones that came so quickly and clearly, she said, "I guess I never really did."

29

Tom

Over the next few days, I tried to digest Teri's story. I shared the experience with friends, breaking down crying every time. "She gave me such a gift, I just can't believe it." Hearing her story made me feel seen––by her and by myself. But I hadn't talked to Teri about any of my experiences with Randy yet.

I called her back later that week and the conversation quickly turned to Vegas. "I remember when Randy called to say your mom was in Texas," she said. "He told me he was going away on a 'boys' weekend' and wanted to know if John could stay with me. That was a red flag," she continued. "In all our years of shared custody, not once did he ask if I could take John. He always fought to keep him away from me."

Hearing this new lie made me sick. "I can't imagine him ever going away on a boys' weekend," I said.

"Well, of course I said it was fine for John to stay with me and then I'll never forget, we were sitting at home that Saturday night when I got a call from my friend, Tom. He lived in Vegas and was pretty upset about what he'd just seen," Teri said.

Who is Tom? What did he see?

"Tom asked me, 'Do you know where your ex-husband is right now?' and I said, 'I thought he was on a boys' weekend.'"

"Well, boys must be a euphemism for young girl, because he's with someone named Ingrid and they are heading out to see Wayne Newton," Tom told Teri.

Tom had come to see Randy at our hotel—I realized now that he was the one who was supposed to have dinner with us—but Teri told me he was so alarmed at seeing Randy and me together, he immediately left the Tropicana and called her instead. "That's when I knew Randy was doing to you what he'd done to me," she said.

Shock waves were pulsing through me. It was one thing to hold my story up against hers, but hearing Teri had done the same was like a bomb going off. And now I understood that Tom, a stranger to me, was equally disturbed. He'd told Teri, "She was too young, even for that guy." Twenty-seven years later, I had never heard such appropriate reactions. It was one of the most affirming moments of my life.

But I had always thought there were only two people who knew I was in Vegas: my stepbrother Sean and my best friend Mita. They were the only people I confided in. Learning that Teri knew and Tom knew was profoundly validating. It meant I *was,* in fact, there. Not that I ever thought I was delusional, but for the others who made me out to be, it was like I finally had corroborators.

These initial feelings became mixed with heartache. I realized Teri didn't do anything with this information. "Did you ever think about telling my mom, or anyone else at the time?" I could tell the question made her uncomfortable as her voice started shaking.

She admitted that she thought about telling my mom, but in the end, she never did. I realized that Teri had been burned too many times to confront Randy again, and I understood. But I was still glad I asked the question, if only to assert that I wished things could have been different.

As we kept talking, Teri casually said, "Tom and I still talk about Vegas to this day."

"You *still* talk to Tom?!" For some reason, it never occurred to me they would still be in touch. We started to wonder collectively if Tom might be willing to talk to me. I had always wanted to know how the trip appeared to someone else but never imagined I would have the chance to ask.

"I can call him now," she said. "I don't imagine why he wouldn't talk to you."

I paced the floor for thirty minutes, wondering if I might get a call from Tom, but it was Teri who called me back.

"Not only does Tom remember seeing Randy in Vegas, after I told him you were looking for more details, he recalled meeting you in the hotel room. He said something felt off before Randy even told him you were his girlfriend."

He said I was his girlfriend?

Teri told me she repeated this detail to Tom, to verify it, and he replied, "Yes, when Ingrid was out of earshot, Randy told me she was his girlfriend."

And here was the real proof. Not just that I was there. But I was there as "his girlfriend."

I didn't make it all up.
I'm not crazy.
I can trust myself.

For so many years, I thought Randy paraded me around *like* a girlfriend. My body knew it, but I never heard him say it, so I couldn't prove it. He did want me to be his girlfriend. He *was* grooming me.

I told Teri I hadn't talked with my mom about Vegas since family therapy in 1991 when she had said, "I believe that you believe those things happened, but I don't believe they did," and Teri's reply surprised me: "I know your mom knows you were in Vegas."

What?

235

"Well, when your mom and Randy still lived at the ranch, I needed to pick something up from their house. Your mom and I were alone that afternoon and ended up having a glass or two of wine. The past just started coming up," Teri said.

Apparently, it was my mom who brought up Vegas. Teri's impression was my mom had some understanding the trip had happened, but she wasn't willing to see the full truth of it. She'd said something to the effect of, "Yes, they went to Las Vegas, but Ingrid was a real pain in the ass in high school."

"It was like she was choosing to look the other way," Teri said.

I instantly felt like a teenager. I could literally hear the sound of my mom's voice, parroting Randy's words. There was a moment of relief at hearing she finally believed Randy had taken me away, but it was closely followed by the recognition she was still making me out as the bad guy.

What am I supposed to do with that? I wondered. When I allowed myself to tap into the tiniest feelings, I became so angry.

This is the real trauma, I thought, or at least a major extension of it. It wasn't just Las Vegas, it was after I got home, the truth never came out and Randy was still pursuing me. When I finally blew the whistle, I turned to the one person I thought might protect me, and instead, she decided I was a *pain in the ass*.

So, I learned how ineffective my hurt and anger were, how unimportant I was. And I began to tuck all my feelings away. They had been tucked away for decades.

Maybe I don't want to know these details, I thought. Maybe being in a "half" relationship with my mom where she makes beautiful, handmade things, and we get together once or twice a year to have a few laughs, is preferable to the reminder of her disregard for me. Because when I looked at the whole relationship, I was starting to see it wasn't that different to the one I had with Randy. I accepted table scraps for a little attention.

The difference was that I couldn't own that truth about my mom like I could with Randy. It was easy to despise him. I didn't need him the way I needed her. I could write off my relationship with Randy, but I couldn't do that with my mom. I was *still* in relationship with her, still needed her and didn't want to lose her.

I shared some of these complicated thoughts with Teri but also knew I needed space to digest it all. "I think I need to go take a nap," I said eventually.

Then Teri said, "You know, you and I were both victims of Randy, but your mom was too." I let her comment wash over me, knowing the truth of it.

"I know she was," I paused before continuing, "she still is. You and I are able to have these conversations, but she still can't face the truth. You and I survived."

We hung up the phone. *My mom knows, but she still doesn't know.* I understood why, but I didn't have a choice to wait anymore, hoping she would come to her senses like I always thought she would. I needed to tell my truth whether she was capable of hearing it or not.

I knew without a doubt what Randy had done. He was grooming me to be his girlfriend. He called me his girlfriend to his friend. He lied to everyone about it and shamed me for his abuses.

Having all of this confirmed had given me more confidence. Everyone related to Randy had given me permission to speak up. The only person left to talk to about it was the one person I wanted to believe me the most, and after my conversation with Teri, I was even more doubtful she would.

30

Walking the Plank

I was forty-three but feeling more and more like my seventeen-year-old-self. As though I was getting ready to make another phone call from the counselor's office. "Hi, Mom, it's me. I really need to talk with you."

I knew intellectually I didn't need my mom's validation, but the child in me still did. I felt more anxious than when the social workers were on their way. At least back then I had some hope she would listen. *So, I'm making myself vulnerable to her again? With pages of our story, thinking maybe this will convince her? And what if it doesn't? I'm just destroyed all over again?*

Those were the questions I was faced with as I started to walk a familiar plank. Except it not only felt like this path could destroy me, it could hurt my little boy. If my mom couldn't face her role in everything, if she couldn't face the truth, I didn't know if we could be in relationship with her anymore.

I was still thinking I would wait to share my book with her only if it ever got published. I imagined I'd send a copy to her best friend, Kathy. Kathy knew Randy, so the details probably wouldn't be too much of a surprise. Kathy had left her own husband after she discovered he was sexually abusing her disabled daughter. I wanted someone with that sort of strength to be a witness to my mom's revisiting of her own past.

But as the days went by, my anxiety rose. It felt like I was sitting on a time bomb and I couldn't continue to exchange pleasantries with my mom on the phone. I couldn't keep it a secret. It didn't matter if I was publishing a book or not, if a publisher made my story "valid" or not. I needed to validate it myself.

I got into my bed and tucked myself under my duvet. Surrounded in white fluffy comfort, I dialed my mom's number. My heartbeat was louder than the ringing I heard on the line. I became so dissociated I was almost shocked when my mom answered. We briefly chatted then I dove in.

"I'm calling because I wanted to talk to you about the writing I've been doing. I know you heard I was maybe writing another book. I've actually almost completed a first draft."

"Oh wow!"

"I know, I've been kind of consumed by it. I'm writing about everything from my alcoholism, to marrying an active alcoholic, to my childhood, and largely … growing up with Randy." And there it was, the subject I'd been avoiding talking to her about for over two decades.

"Oh. Well, it should be interesting," she said, a little too cheerfully.

"Yeah, it is interesting for sure. I've talked to Stacy, Sean, and John but I wanted to give you an opportunity to have a voice as well. I had no intentions of writing it. But something happened for me...," I started to cry, "...after Randy died. I felt like I finally had a voice again. I was flooded with memories that were waking me in the middle of the night, having to write them down."

She was quiet and it felt like the floodgates had opened so I kept going.

"I've honestly felt freer since he passed. And I'm tired of having his version of the story be the only one. I need to tell my side. You and I have not talked about any of this since I was still in high school, and I guess I want to give you an opportunity from this place in your life to tell me what you understand about that time."

"Well..." There was a long pause. "I'd have to think about it some. I don't know what to say right now."

I knew she wasn't expecting this, that she felt overwhelmed. I told her how I was originally thinking I would just send her the book when it was finished, but didn't want to ambush her with an entire text. "I don't know what depth of conversation you and I will ever have about it, but I don't feel okay with the elephant in the room anymore."

Caution creeping into her voice, she replied, "I can understand that. And I can understand where you are coming from. It's just something that I don't feel comfortable about. I don't know if I want to bring up all those *feelings* in me."

I told her that never talking about it was starting to feel dishonest to me and making me feel far away from her. And that maybe, for the first time, we could have a different relationship now that Randy was gone—a closer one, but not unless we acknowledged what happened.

The more we talked, the more I felt like I was trying to swim against a current of polite but stubborn resistance. She kept saying, "I understand … if that's what you feel you need to do… if it makes you feel better, then I suppose that's good…" Never once getting in the water with me, never acknowledging that anything I was saying was real.

I finally said, "I've been holding a lot of hurt for a long time because nobody else could see it, witness it, and believe it. And I'm finally saying *this is real.* It happened. It's pretty fucked up and I'm not going to keep it a secret anymore. At some point, I need us to address things more directly. At least that's my hope. Why don't you think about it."

She agreed and we hung up. I let out a long breath I didn't know I'd been holding. I felt a little lighter and proud of myself for being so bold.

But our second phone call wasn't any more productive. My mom seemed even more determined to put off any hard conversations, saying, "My psyche is pretty fragile right now, Ingrid. I've had a hard time getting through this last year and I just don't know if can even go there right now. This is stuff that happened twenty-five years ago and I understand that you need to do what you need to do, but I don't know that I'm ready."

I told her yes, for twenty-five years I'd been holding in my side of the story, twenty-five years of feeling like I wasn't believed, and I just couldn't do it anymore. That if she were to maintain that none of it ever happened, I would have a really hard time with that.

"I can't do anything about the past. I can only do something about today and tomorrow," was her answer. Then she started to cry. "I love you very much…" She paused for a long time, her voice so shaky and soft she was barely able to finish. "I hope that we can still have a halfway decent relationship. And maybe somewhere down the road. But I just can't do it now."

I told her I understood, and that for now, I would just keep writing until the time came when she felt ready to talk about it. She took another long pause and said, "Well, I'll probably try and go to yoga this afternoon. I haven't done anything like that in weeks, and I really need it."

"Well, that sounds like a good idea, Mom …" I said.

31

Unfinished Business

I initially felt some relief after that conversation with my mom. At least I wasn't keeping my writing a secret. Then I returned to the comfort of my longing: *Maybe one day she'll face the truth.* I carried that hope around like a time capsule for three and a half years while life marched on.

We entered a global pandemic and Henry graduated kindergarten. My dad's health declined and he passed away. As we'd done for decades, conversations with my mom were a few times a month and related to comfortable topics in the present tense. I would occasionally feel her support, but mostly the same emotional distance.

The longer Randy had been gone, the more my mom seemed to revere him. Yancey and I didn't see family for a long while due to Covid, but we finally made it back to Colorado. My mom had moved to Rifle to live with her friend Kathy. My brother Josh moved there too and we spent several days with them in the mountains.

As my mom showed me to her bedroom, where Yancey and I were meant to sleep, it was like walking into Randy's shrine. The old posters that used to hang above his piano were looming large over her bed. The sight of his things made my skin crawl, but I didn't say a word. At least not to my mom.

We took family photos, ate lovely meals, and played Uno as a family. My mom drank in the evenings, seemed annoyed that Henry didn't show her love the way she wanted, and I felt the same way I always had——like this was an obligation. Like my mom didn't know me at all, but this was what it looked like to be a "good daughter." You show up. You accept your mother's limitations, privilege her wounds. You understand that she's doing the best she can. Only now I felt angry about it.

I had spent years of my life compiling evidence, getting clarity and seeking support from anyone who would listen. My commitment to healing had become a full-time job and I *was* healing. But this relationship was feeling more and more like a stumbling block.

I wasn't ready to address any of this on that visit. *Just finish the book.* I knew when I had to confront her in order to move forward with publishing, I would do it. And likely not a moment sooner.

***

It was April of 2022 and I was sitting at my kitchen table on a Monday night when I saw a message from Facebook pop up. Henry was asleep and Yancey was watching TV on the couch.

"I wish I never read your book, because I have no respect for your mom now."

It was from my mom's friend and roommate, Kathy. I had sent her a copy of my manuscript, along with other family and friends who were in the book. I was getting closer to finishing and needed to see if anyone had strong objections or wanted to change their name. I was also hoping Kathy could be a bridge of understanding between my mom and I. We talked about my book when I was in Colorado and Kathy believed me. She and I sat in tears in her bathroom while my mom was at the doctor. "I'll do whatever I can to help your mom see the truth," she'd said.

Seeing her message, a knot instantly formed in my stomach. It never occurred to me this might happen. I had been so nervous about the wrath that could come for me, I didn't see the possibility that my mom might face her own consequences. *Oh no, this is going in the wrong direction.*

"I just can't understand how she didn't advocate for you," she continued. "Whenever I bring it up, she just screams that you are a liar. She won't even acknowledge it and it really bothers me. Whenever we have a conversation about it, she wakes up the next day like nothing happened. Just like in the book. Head in the sand. I'm so sorry."

The knot turned to nausea. "Yancey," I said, "can you please come here?" As I read him Kathy's message, I started to cry as though I were choking. Coughing tears that had been lodged in my throat like a dam had just broken. *I can't believe it. She's screaming that I'm a liar.*

Yancey hugged me and I actually let him. I was stunned, fighting to figure this all out, like a math problem my life depended on. Whatever I had perceived as a window of ownership in that conversation with my mom was clearly a closed door. It was never going to open. I felt forced to see something I had never seen this clearly. I had always looked at my mother's denial as the issue, but I was the one with blinders on. It was humiliating.

"If she still thinks I'm a liar, I can't be in relationship with her anymore," I responded to Kathy, and I meant it. I was surprised how much I meant it. It didn't feel like a choice, as though my body was revolting and letting me know it would not stand for this one minute longer. I could not stand in front of a locked door, hoping my sanity, peace, relief would be set free if only my mother would open it.

"I'm in shock," I told Yancey. He and I talked about how he had seen me in this place so many times. How I responded to each and every terrible incident in my life as though it were isolated. We marveled at my ability to give everyone the benefit of the doubt—to believe in the power and possibility of change—my *hope* had been a deterrent to my ever seeing the truth.

But how is anyone supposed to comprehend that their mother abandoned them? The feelings that accompanied such a blow were too devastating for words, but I was beginning to feel them, and a part of me knew it was better than all of my waiting. Because in the waiting, *I was doing it again.* I was abandoning myself.

I went numb and curled up on the couch next to Yancey. We tucked ourselves under a weighted blanket and watched mindless TV before going to bed. When I woke up early the next morning, I composed a text to my mom. It flew out of me without too much thought but it said everything. Then I did not send it. I wanted to sit with it. I wanted to know what it would feel like to say goodbye to my mom. To feel the weight of that decision, for myself and my family.

Initially, I noticed some relief. I was fiercely advocating for myself and that felt like the right thing to do. I felt my strength. I thought of all the obligatory calls and visits and the idea of never doing that again was liberating. I felt more authentic.

I also experienced an instantaneous new level of love for my son. As though cutting off from the destructive way my mom saw me allowed me to stop seeing him through a judgmental lens. *I had the capacity to be a better mom.*

I realized I didn't have to be all things to all people. I could disappoint people. I could make mistakes. Like my perfectionism could finally bugger off. It felt profound. I didn't have to try so damn hard all the time. *I surrender!*

These felt like truths in my bones, ones I'd never felt this deeply. My body was giving me so much feedback that I was moving in the right direction, I couldn't ignore it. But it also couldn't protect me from the harsh reality of the big picture. The text I had composed to my mom felt like another break-up, a divorce, a death. *I can't believe it's come to this; it's really ending.*

The heartbreak was torture, knowing I never really had my mother to begin with. Depression was coming. I could taste it. The heaviness and exhaustion. Anger too. I could feel its heat.

I was lying in bed a couple of days after Kathy's message and I couldn't sleep—tossing and turning, the tears starting to come. I didn't want to cry. *Please don't cry. Please don't feel this, it's too much, I can't do it.*

I wanted to tell Yancey what was going on, but I couldn't. The kid in me who saw that her mother had given up on her was too embarrassed. I felt worthless, even with the person I knew loved me the most. I felt *gross.*

I went to the bathroom and sat in the dark, my body on the cold toilet seat and my face in my hands. *This is so awful,* I cried as I rocked back and forth, the sobs relentless.

A flash of anger came. *What was the point of all of this?* The clarity I had gained through my writing, sharing and healing—for this? *What the fuck have I done?* My hopelessness was like a blackout. Deep and dark, unable to see, my tears kept falling. *I don't have any purpose or meaning. I don't want to be a therapist. I don't want to kill myself, but it would be okay if I died.*

Decades of devastation were coming for me. Years of pent-up pain. I cried like this for over an hour, until I was too tired to weep. The feelings were still with me, but all my energy was gone. I crawled back to bed, feeling gravely alone.

The next morning, I told Yancey what had happened. The look on his face, where he felt so much sadness but didn't know how to say it, shattered me. I knew he was coming from a loving place, but I couldn't feel it. I only felt pathetic and that made me feel everything all over again. *I am discardable. I'm not worth it. Not even my own mother could love me.*

And then, somehow, we got Henry ready for school, and I showed up for six clients over Zoom. I did what I had always done, said the things I needed to hear. Felt hope I needed to feel—not the hope that someone else might change, but that I could feel better even when they didn't.

I had to take my own advice and lean into any self-care that felt remotely possible. I took hot baths. I listened to music. I let myself be in disarray, ordering more takeout, eating more ice cream, only wearing sweatpants.

One week after I received Kathy's message, I was volunteering at Henry's school. I had been reading to the kids in his class every Monday, and on that day, I saw Henry receive an award. They announced his name over the loud speaker and it was amazing to witness his face, embarrassed but smiling so big. *That's my boy.*

I left the school thinking I might go for a hike. It was a beautiful day and I'd been turning to nature as a powerful resource. The sun on my face felt healing. The trees helped me breathe. Walking was helping me process everything.

But as I arrived at my car, I opened my phone and saw comments my mom had made on my personal Facebook page. Lovely comments, ones you would imagine a grandmother to make. But they just made me angry. *She can't keep pretending to be loving when she's screaming that I'm a liar.* I opened the message I had written for my mom a week earlier and hit send.

> Staying in relationship with you, knowing you believe I'm manipulative - has kept me from healing - from ever being my true self. I am finally choosing to love myself no matter what

you or anyone else thinks of me. I never wanted it to come to this. But I can no longer have you in my life while you hold Randy in such esteem and continue to view me as delusional. It doesn't feel like a choice anymore. It feels like I should have done this a long time ago…

I didn't want to have another conversation. I didn't want to hear her defense, or allow anything to change my mind. I just wanted it to be done.

As I re-read the message, I felt dizzy. I couldn't think straight, but suddenly realized it was Randy's birthday. I couldn't believe I sent that text on his birthday.

I took some deeper breaths and started my car, not knowing where I was going. I needed food, so when I saw McDonald's a few blocks away, I went through the drive-through.

"Are you still serving breakfast?" *I just told my mom she can't be in my life.* "Okay, great. I'll have an Egg McMuffin, please." *What is happening?*

I sat in the parking lot, staring at the black trash bins across the alley. It was trash day. I was sitting in a fast food parking lot, washing hash browns down with orange juice. *This is not my life.*

As I felt a little less dissociated, I couldn't believe what I was feeling: It was hope. *What is wrong with me?!*

252

I hated that hope was still the first thing to rise. But I couldn't deny it, and it was sitting right next to its best friend, guilt. In a distant third was self-trust and something like feeling proud of myself. At least I wasn't wavering that this was the right thing to do.

I texted Yancey, knowing he was knee-deep at work. I texted some friends. Then I felt paralyzed again. My thoughts turned to Josh. *I don't think he'll understand.* He was so close to our mom and I wondered if I would lose him, too.

One of my friends responded. She wondered if I could connect with my therapist or sponsor. I wasn't currently in therapy and meetings had taken a backseat in the pandemic. But I knew her instincts were right. Although we hadn't connected in a while, I texted Bill.

He wrote me back immediately and then I drove forty minutes to a café in the valley where we had sat many times before. This was where he helped me through my divorce. Where he supported my interest in Yancey. Sitting across from Bill, it was all settling in. I was settling in. As he'd always done, Bill validated my experience. He helped me believe I was worth taking care of, no matter the cost. We gave each other a big hug as we walked back towards my car and then it was time for me to pick Henry up from school.

My mom didn't text back immediately, an hour later, or even that same evening. However, my stepbrother John told me she'd sent him a text that night. Their annual "raising a glass to Randy" for his birthday message. The contrast was striking. Right as I told my mom she was losing me by choosing Randy, she was celebrating him.

The next day, I started to wonder whether she'd received my text at all when I saw a message on my phone.

> Dear Ingrid, I am so sorry. Hope your book helps you heal. Personally I choose to not live in the past. I can not change it. Everyone makes mistakes. I am sorry for mine. I love and care about you and your family. I pray for you every night. Love Mom.

On the surface, some of it seemed loving. But I turned my attention away from her words and towards their impact. I asked myself questions I might have asked a client:

Do I feel seen, heard or respected? *No.*

Do I feel understood or validated? *No.*

Do I feel like she wants to make things right? *No.*

Do I feel overridden, blamed, shamed or manipulated? *Yes.*

When I answered these questions, it was clear. My mom was saying nothing at all in her message. I'd never heard her mention a single "mistake" she claimed she was sorry for. Was it when she abandoned me thirty years ago, or was it last week when she called me a liar?

I noticed her comment about "not living in the past." It's one trauma survivors get all the time and it's a gross misrepresentation of trauma. Being traumatized is not a choice. Trauma is not something that happened "back then," it's not in the past at all. It's an ongoing experience of feeling deeply unsafe and terrorized, over and over, in the present moment.

I tried to leave the past in the past in a million ways, but the past never left me. It's like a thread was woven deeply into my body, stitching past and present together until I couldn't decipher which was which.

My mom didn't understand that; it's as though she saw trauma as a moral failing. But we can't forgive trauma into submission. We can't out-think, run, pray, talk, or good-deed it away. That's just friendly-looking avoidance and I couldn't avoid it anymore. And I couldn't continue trying to heal on my own, never bothering or burdening her.

I kept thinking about Henry, wondering what was best for him. I used to worry I would do him a disservice if I "took his grandmother away," but that's not what happened. I was unplugging from the source of my pain so I didn't hand its legacy to him. I found myself returning to the same conclusion: If I felt about Henry the way my mom felt about me, *I would want him to cut me out of his life.*

My mother's need to stay in denial was understandable. She would have to admit her entire life was a lie, that she put me in harm's way, left me there, and then blamed me for it. But understanding *why* she did it didn't mean I needed to stay in relationship.

I finally felt the full impact of my mother and if I *had* to choose, I would rather have me in my life than her in my life. What a horrible choice, but I was making it, the week of Mother's Day. Thirty years later, I could recall that Mother's Day brunch when I felt like numbness and denial were easier and declare with certainty: they are not. With a mix of sadness and self-respect I could say, *Happy Mother's Day* to me. I was breaking a cycle, doing the brave and brutal work of healing trauma.

I had been a "good girl" for decades. I tried to be in acceptance, living with my mother's alcoholism and denial, connecting with the best parts of her, thinking they were enough. What I never understood was how that kept me in harm's way. I had to leave the most important parts of myself at the door, never able to claim them as my own. I never realized that staying in relationship to a mother who saw me as broken made me believe I actually was.

32

Finding My Voice

My mom hasn't changed since my writing first emerged, but something *has* fundamentally shifted. It didn't happen all at once, but I eventually noticed I didn't need her to believe me in the way I always had. I realized for the first time in a very long time, *I believed me.*

I had spent so many painful years hoping the people who had hurt me would help me. I thought they *could.* I thought they held the keys to my freedom. But as I reclaimed my story, I saw how I was doing the work I had always wanted them to do. I had to be the one to save me.

The more solid I felt about everything that happened, the less ashamed I became. I could see myself more clearly, like the Chevron sign on Beverly Boulevard with its vibrant blues and reds. Like hundreds of negative filters had been lifted from my eyes, I could see a larger storyline. One I'd never seen in all my personal therapy, formal education, ongoing training: I have unresolved, complex trauma. In fact, I have Complex PTSD.

I didn't know this for the first few years I was writing this book. I needed to feel safe enough, from the privacy of my own MacBook, sitting in my house, to really *see*. The writing became an unfiltered way for me to experience things in black and white, to put them in context, and then observe them from a therapist's perspective. I had to linger a long time over each sentence, noticing how it started on the surface, but called to me to drill down. I needed to retrace my own steps, go back and give myself permission to feel, to see what I saw, and to regain the parts of me that were left behind.

My need to create a coherent narrative of my life—for the book's sake, for the reader's sake—helped me to keep going every time I wanted to stop. It's like I dropped my internal world into this external container that provided just enough distance and safety, and then it kept pulling me into clarity, into a fuller existence, into healing.

Before I was struck with the urgency to revisit my past, I just thought I was broken. But my story became my personal textbook. By engaging with it in the present moment, with some psychological knowledge as a tether, I could finally see the through line. And what I saw was obvious: All the ways I had coped: my perfectionism, people-pleasing, addictions, denial, codependency, striving, relationships with narcissists … were all trauma responses.

I started to realize *This is what complex trauma looks like*. It can look like a successful woman who's been sober for twenty-six years, who has a beautiful family … and yet she's still saddled with so much self-doubt about the truth of her own life. She's still anxious and ashamed, worried she's going to "get in trouble," still tolerating abusive behavior. Somewhere in there, I started to see these things as *common* trauma responses. And from this lens, it was abundantly clear that trauma had taken a hold of me early on and never let me go.

In some ways, my confusion was not just my own. While I kept beating back my "flaws," telling myself my childhood *wasn't that bad*, the larger mental health community was in a decades-long debate. Even though Dr. Bessel van der Kolk was talking about developmental trauma (now synonymous with complex trauma) in my 2004 training, we have yet to formally adopt a diagnosis in the United States.

It was only recently that the World Health Organization named Complex PTSD (CPTSD) in its *International Classification of Diseases, 11th Revision*. This was in 2018, the same year I started putting pieces of my own life into context, making these connections myself.

And yet, these revelations were like the tip of an iceberg. Even with all of this knowledge, I still didn't quite believe it. Self-gaslighting is a *force*. And healing from trauma is a process. It's never linear, where we get insights in sequential order that continually build on one another. It looks like three steps forward, four backwards, two to the side... It's lopsided, circuitous, and looks different for every individual.

In my process, the next step of healing meant going on social media. I reluctantly started a professional profile on Instagram and began searching for hashtags. I'd never done this before and surprised myself by looking up #complextrauma. I wasn't ready to say, *I'm a trauma survivor*, but the necessity of a hashtag made me choose that one.

Within moments of searching, I saw posts for #traumasurvivor and #narcissisticparent and my life was forever changed. *These are my people!* The memes and tiny bits of digestible information, spoken in such a raw and undiluted fashion spoke to my soul. I felt like I'd stumbled into a parallel universe that carried all the answers I was looking for my entire life.

I was reminded of going to AA and comparing that experience with what I had learned in graduate school about addiction. In my view, there is no theory, diagnosis or therapy that can replace the power of shared experience. The community piece is a major source of understanding and healing. Survivors speak about trauma from the gut, from the heart, where the hurt lives, and I identified with just about everything that crossed my feed.

I could finally see how I had been stuck in a trauma response for decades and it just seemed normal. I could understand how I never "got over it" with traditional psychotherapy or my recovery from addiction. Trying to practice "moving on" or "forgiveness" without deeper healing would have left me abandoned by the one person who could have saved me: myself. I couldn't move on until I had actually processed and integrated everything that had happened. I couldn't move on until I could see how I was still in my own way.

I started creating content, personal memes related to narcissistic abuse, and it was terrifying. I had written pages of material on this subject, but it was sitting on my computer. I had shared it in classes and writing groups, but never like *this*. I was posting as a psychologist, but largely as a *survivor*, in public. I was exposing secrets, challenging old narratives and challenging myself. It was equal parts freeing and petrifying. Like I couldn't wait to jump, but was certain I was about to splat on the concrete. I was loving the creativity, but it was *scary*. Every time.

Instagram became a place for me to practice having a voice. It was an extension of my writing, which up until that point was the method of my healing. I had faced so much of my shame and made others face reality with me. I had become relentless in my need to validate my experience, to validate me. I was doing the very thing I had been afraid of doing for so long, telling the truth.

Then Instagram made a big shift, away from static memes, towards short-form video content. Once again, I was reluctant. I couldn't imagine putting my actual face on this material. But the performer in me loved the creativity and the opportunity to bring humor to such heavy topics.

One day I saw a traditional makeup tutorial and thought, *What if I did a makeup tutorial on complex trauma?* I could see the whole thing in my mind and grabbed my makeup and computer before I could talk myself out of it. I recorded the video in one take and thought it was absurd, but hilarious. So, I posted it. Then I learned how to lip sync, adding my spin on trauma and narcissistic abuse to other people's audio. I was cracking myself up thinking, *I am about to tank my career, but I'm having so much fun!*

I was being all of me in one place at the same time and it was liberating. And the more I posted, the more feedback I received. I never got validation from the places I always wanted, but I was getting it now. It made me reflect on how we can stay stuck in a small circle, thinking all our needs must be met in that patch of real estate. Maybe our needs can't be met in our family of origin, our immediate friend group, our home town ... but that doesn't mean we can't get our needs met. Sometimes, when we feel stuck, we just need to widen our circle.

All the comments and messages of resonance and gratitude were uplifting. They were coming from all over the world. And the accounts I started following were blowing my mind with their courage and wisdom. This was the community I had been missing and I didn't even know it. A place where I was a therapist, a performer, a survivor, and I was allowed to have fun. I was helping other people but I was also helping myself, without having to hide.

I started to see the importance of transparency as a psychologist or anyone in the helping professions. How can we help others heal from an antiquated, binary, broken or healed paradigm if we aren't willing to admit that we don't have it all figured out? I know how compelling it is to think someone has all the answers, that they've transcended the human condition. And I know how it feels to come up short when I don't meet that unrealistic expectation. Appearing fully cooked is a great marketing tool, but we are selling a fantasy.

The revelations I was having on social media about trauma were equally matched by what I was learning about narcissism. I never saw Randy's behavior through the lens of narcissistic traits, he was just *Randy*. I didn't know I grew up in a fog of gaslighting, I just thought I was confused about the extent to which he was grooming me. Once I could own that language, it put all of the stories that had flooded my brain into context. Like another layer of tracing paper, mapping out perfectly over what I'd written. Phrases like love-bombing, future faking, smear campaigns, and scapegoat all became personal to me and validated my experiences even more.

My puzzle was complete when I saw my experiences in these fuller contexts. I'd been rummaging through other puzzle boxes all my life, looking for the perfect fit, but this was it. When I knew what was "wrong," I could lean deeper into recovery. Nowhere in all my training had I heard, "Befriend your abuser, it's the path to freedom! Put all of your worth and value into a narcissist's hands!" I joke, but realizing I was a trauma survivor gave me permission to let these old, subconscious strategies go. I could start setting healthier boundaries. I sought other forms of trauma therapy like EMDR (Eye Movement Desensitization and Reprocessing) and IFS (Internal Family Systems).

Today, if someone said to me: "I don't believe you. You're a liar. You made the whole thing up," I would be appalled. I can't imagine any scenario where I would say this to another human being and I will never say it to myself again. I am finally a witness to my own pain. I can respond to my feelings with permission, compassion and validation.

Rather than reclaiming my voice, I saw it was never taken from me. My voice isn't something I have to fight for, it's mine. This is my song and as I sing it, I can set my own record straight. I can turn the tables. Just because "they" could never see me, I don't have to be invisible. I wrote my way to a new ending that allowed me to be seen and heard, even if it was only by me.

Epilogue

Tiny Magic

I am changed by this process. If I were to begin writing this book today, I would not be able to recall the memories that came so forcefully and with such vivid detail. They are not in my present tense awareness anymore. They are finally in the past, still my memories—my experiences—but it feels as though they belong to me more than I belong to them.

As my trauma responses are receding, a fuller self is emerging. In some ways, I am feeling more myself than I ever have. I'm excited to get to know this person, and sad that she is just coming into focus as a forty-seven-year-old woman.

As I continue to heal, I'm flipping the old script. I'm starting from a place of knowing I'm a whole and worthy person, not presupposing that I'm *wrong*. In this process, it's like I get to own all the beautiful parts of me for the first time. We don't just feel and own all of our pain, we get to feel and own all of our goodness too. All the accomplishments and pieces of me I couldn't really see or believe, I get to feel them, own them: *Hell yes, I did all those things!* I can feel proud, strong, creative, kind, and smart.

But I am aware that healing is going to be lifelong. There isn't a place where we go, "Phew! I did it. Mission complete." There's just our ongoing, sometimes messy, sometimes beautiful existence. And somewhere in there, somewhere in all of that is *me*. Not outside of it, fully recovered, standing on a mountain top. Not having arrived at some magical destination. I see now that the giant and elusive thing I always wanted for myself has actually been coming in a million tiny moments every step along the way, and it's continuing even now.

That training with van der Kolk, my sobriety, therapy, and eventually each word I wrote for this book, every interview I conducted, all the insight, determination, I can see now that tiny magic was happening. All the moments that led up to my ability to write this truth were more powerful than some external celebration or culmination of it.

My whole life I had been looking for a goddammed explosion. I'm not sure if that's "alcoholic thinking" or just being human, but I lived in that longing. Waiting for the enormous, undeniable victory over my brokenness. And this striving obscured the healing that was happening at every turn.

Right now, as I write these words, my darling husband is taking a nap and Henry is watching cartoons. We went to a creek this morning and Henry caught some frogs. We are all here, each doing our own quiet thing. This is the moment I've been waiting for. This is the answered prayer and I can tap into this beautiful reality anytime I want.

Maybe none of my therapists could have helped me all those years ago, because they couldn't see it any clearer than I could. Maybe I had to become my own therapist, and that is both magical and heartbreaking. Just like everything else.

Maybe I wanted to die in my bathroom that night because a part of me was, in fact, dying: the parts of me that needed to die, the parts that were a lie, the trauma responses I thought were me. And when I felt that intense loss, it allowed new parts to grow. My growth was in my conscious awareness that my needs were never met. When I felt that truth, my body could stop engaging in patterns where my needs would never be met, and I could feel safer than I ever had before.

I always knew what happened and I knew I felt stuck; it was the connective tissue that was missing. In order to connect the dots, I had to let go of the fantasy that it wasn't that bad. Because it was. I had to feel the truth of how I wasn't taken care of. This feeling, this grief, is why I believe that healing trauma is some of the hardest work. It can feel more devastating than the wound itself. It makes me understand why I wanted my mom to be the connective tissue. Getting repair is a lot easier than living with unprocessed pain. But never getting it doesn't have to be the stumbling block I always thought it was.

As I wake Henry up every morning, I feel into myself before I walk in his room, knowing that he is reading my nervous system whether I am conscious of it or not. He is reading how I feel about myself, how I feel about him, and if I don't double down on seeing myself from a place of love, he will get the message that we both aren't worth it.

I wanted to do this work for my mom. I often wished I could know what her childhood was really like, what wounds she was unconsciously carrying and repeating. But those specifics wouldn't help me to heal her—I couldn't do her work for her no matter how hard I tried.

Knowing the specifics of what happened to any of us isn't the answer to our healing. Many people will never know the specifics of their story because they were in a state of dissociation while it unfolded. It was helpful to have my experiences validated, no question. But there's a reason I knew I had to validate them to begin with: I knew what was true. I knew that I had been invalidated. And my fierce determination to get whatever I needed in order to believe and validate myself was the answer.

The clues to complex trauma aren't so much in our story as they are in our present-day symptoms. And we don't need to have PTSD to have symptoms. We are all imprinted, we all have a nervous system. We are all relational beings, impacting one another, being impacted. The patterns I relived and repeated, those were the signs, the clues that ultimately led me to my truth.

I now have a deep commitment to breaking the cycle—in me and in my family. I am writing a new story. One where I won't tolerate being discarded. Where I live a sober life and my son will never see his mother drink, or drive drunk, or blindly rage. I will listen to him. I will respect where he is coming from. I will do it imperfectly, but I will apologize when I am wrong.

This is my story. The one Randy could never take from me. My mom doesn't hold the key to this happiness, I do.

I was never broken. I was a perfectly functioning human being, reacting to the traumatic experiences of my childhood exactly the way I was meant to survive them. Then I sought out and discovered friendships, healers, insights, programs, hikes, heart-shaped clouds in the sky … healing that poured through me and onto others in a way that has given me joy and purpose.

All that has happened and is still happening.
This is me.
Here I am.
My whole story.
Unfolding, imperfect, healing, and glorious.

Glossary

While there are many different clinical lenses with which to view my story, what follows are some terms that felt personally relevant once I put my experiences in the context of narcissism and complex trauma. I hope they serve as a guide in furthering your own understanding and healing.

Complex Trauma:

Complex trauma refers to repeated exposure to traumatic events, relational in nature, and the long-terms effects of that exposure.

Complex PTSD (CPTSD):

Complex PTSD shares similar criteria with PTSD, including:

- Reexperiencing traumatic events (nightmares, unwanted memories, flashbacks)

- Avoidance of traumatic reminders (people, places, feelings, thoughts)
- A persistent sense of current threat (hypervigilance)

But it extends beyond these to include:

- Difficulty regulating emotions
- Negative self-concept
- Disturbances in relationships (typically associated with sustained, repeated, or multiple forms of traumatic exposure)

With complex trauma, there is a distortion in a person's core sense of self. Additionally, PTSD is often related to a single event, whereas CPTSD includes repeated traumatic events, often in childhood.

Complex Trauma is used interchangeably with *developmental trauma* and *relational trauma*.

Emotional Flashbacks:

A flashback is when we reexperience a traumatic event as if it is happening in the present moment.

Pete Walker, a psychotherapist who specializes in complex trauma, refers to emotional flashbacks as "sudden and often prolonged regressions ('amygdala hijackings') to the frightening and abandoned feeling-states of childhood."

Sometimes we can identify a specific external trigger, sometimes flashbacks are related to our physical state, and sometimes they happen out of the blue.

My repeated experience of feeling like I'm about to "get in trouble," is an example of an emotional flashback.

Fawning Trauma Response:

Fawning is a trauma response. Pete Walker coined the term *fawning* and believes it is at the core of codependent behavior. I prefer the term fawning to "codependency" as it is rooted in a deeper understanding of trauma and feels less stigmatized.

Fawning is a common response to complex trauma, tapping into someone's mood and adapting to their needs. It occurs when we mirror or merge with another in order to avoid conflict and find safety, when we lack assertiveness and relinquish healthy boundaries.

Fawners often grew up in abusive households or have at least one parent with high narcissistic traits. In childhood, they were shamed out of developing a healthy sense of self and learned to privilege their abuser's needs.

It's important to remember that fawning is an unconscious survival strategy. And at the same time, it causes the person doing it to abandon their own needs, thereby reinforcing their wounding.

Because survival goes hand-in-hand with being exploited, fawners are often repeatedly drawn to people who exploit them. This repetition compulsion, or trauma reenactment, makes sense in the lens of fawning because safety and exploitation have become fused.

In addition to repeating this fawning pattern with people with narcissistic traits, it is not uncommon to bring fawning tendencies to any relationship, threatening or not.

Gaslighting:

From the 1944 film, *Gaslight*, the term gaslighting is a colloquialism for psychological abuse that is designed to make someone question their reality. People who gaslight seek power and control through what is typically a long-term abuse strategy including deflection, denial, withholding, trivializing, lying and questioning the victim's memory.

Self-Gaslighting (Internalized Gaslighting):

Self-gaslighting is a symptom of being gaslit, where the victim continues to question their reality and gaslights themselves based on the original manipulation. It can sound like:

"Maybe it wasn't that bad."

"I didn't experience 'real' trauma."

"If I were a stronger or more spiritual person, I wouldn't feel this way."

"He didn't actually mean what I thought he meant."

"She didn't believe me because I'm not worth believing."

"I should be over this by now."
"I'm being too sensitive and probably overreacting."

One of the insidious things about gaslighting and self-gaslighting is their invisible nature, making them hard to identify.

Signs of being gaslit: questioning yourself, ruminating about character flaws you have been accused of, confused about "what is real," making excuses for the abuser's behavior.

People who have been gaslit don't just question specific events, they tend to start questioning everything. The feeling that they can't trust themselves becomes generalized.

Invalidating Environment:

The environment we grow up in shapes who we are and our experiences. An invalidating environment is one in which important people communicate, directly or indirectly, that we are wrong or invisible. Like other forms of abuse, childhood invalidation can create severe, long-term emotional dysregulation. This happens when healthy emotional reactions are ignored, trivialized, or judged as shameful. When children are punished for "over-reacting" or blamed for their abuse. Gaslighting is a form of invalidation.

According to Marsha Linehan, the creator of Dialectical Behavior Therapy (DBT), the invalidating environment is a key part of how people develop borderline personality disorder (BPD). While I do not meet the criteria for BPD, there is overlap between BPD and C-PTSD, and my experiences of pervasive childhood invalidation are consistent with Dr. Linehan's theory.

Similar to DBT, much of my healing process was about counteracting my childhood invalidation, by developing self-trust and embracing my emotions—largely by thoroughly and openly acknowledging the facts of my traumatic events, and by validating, allowing, and experiencing my feelings.

Narcissistic Abuse:

Narcissistic Abuse is a colloquialism used by survivors to describe emotional and psychological abuse carried out by someone with high narcissistic traits.

Narcissism falls on a spectrum, and most people fall somewhere on it. However, narcissistic abuse is related to people with very high narcissistic traits or Narcissistic Personality Disorder (NPD) that employ the abuse tactics listed under *Narcissistic Abuse Tactics* below.

NPD can often go undiagnosed because the person with the disorder does not seek treatment. The disorder is ego-syntonic in that it presents in alignment with the person's values and needs.

Most often, it is survivors of narcissistic abuse who end up seeking treatment, or researching the personality disorder in an attempt to put their experiences in context.

My intention is not to demonize a mental health disorder by using the term narcissistic abuse. As I understand it, narcissism is also often born of abuse. However, it is my opinion that emotional and psychological abuse in the hands of someone with high narcissist traits, or NPD, is a specific problem given the nature of the disorder (entitlement, lack of empathy, or remorse). I also understand that not all people with high narcissist traits are abusers and not all abusers have NPD. I believe my stepfather was both.

In my process, I had to name narcissism in order to begin deeper healing. I believe many survivors have been underserved in the mental health community, living with undiagnosed C-PTSD as a result of narcissistic abuse, and that naming the abuse specifically is a major piece of recovery. In this way, the language of narcissism is for the survivor. We needed the label in order to see everything in context, to validate the confusion, to break free from the gaslighting, often in community with other survivors.

Narcissistic Abuse Tactics:

While not exhaustive, the following abuse tactics are often exhibited by people with high narcissistic traits:

Verbal abuse, physical abuse, isolation, lying, control, denial, future faking (talking about an idyllic future in order to bond or manipulate), the silent treatment, stalking, hoovering (manipulation tactic designed to reel a victim in when they have tried to leave), love bombing (gifts and flattery used as manipulation, to gain power over and make someone feel indebted), smear campaigns and gaslighting.

Narcissistic Family System:

There tends to be common roles in narcissistic family systems. Based on the five people who lived in my house growing up they are as follows:

Scapegoat: I was (one of) the scapegoats in my family. The scapegoat is the person who takes the blame. They are often the truth-tellers about the family's dysfunction.

Golden Child: This was my stepbrother John. The golden child is the opposite of the scapegoat, the target of praise and adoration. This person can do no wrong in the eyes of the narcissist.

The Enabler/Orbiter: This was my mother. The enabler's life revolves around the narcissist, keeping the marriage intact. The enabler buys into the narcissist's lies and doesn't question their authority.

Sometimes referred to as "secondary abusers" because their behavior enables the primary abuse.

The Lost Child: This was my brother Josh. The lost child blends into the background, is quiet, can become a loner. They don't bother getting upset and seem withdrawn.

Narcissistic Personality Disorder (NPD):

The American Psychological Association defines NPD as a personality disorder with the following characteristics:
(a) a long-standing pattern of grandiose self-importance and an exaggerated sense of talent and achievements;
(b) fantasies of unlimited sex, power, brilliance, or beauty;
(c) an exhibitionistic need for attention and admiration;
(d) either cool indifference or feelings of rage, humiliation, or emptiness as a response to criticism, indifference, or defeat; and
(e) various interpersonal disturbances, such as feeling entitled to special favors, taking advantage of others, and inability to empathize with the feelings of others.

Narcissistic Traits:

Narcissism falls on a spectrum and only a small percentage of people meet the full criteria for NPD. However, others might have a combination of the following narcissistic traits, with or without a diagnosis:

Feels superior to others
Controlling and manipulative
Need for excessive attention/admiration
Entitlement
Profoundly selfish
Lacks a core sense of self
Projects their shame and shortcomings onto others
Exploitative
Arrogant
Overestimates personal talents and achievements
Lacks empathy

Toxic Shame:

A core symptom of complex trauma, toxic shame is feeling fundamentally flawed, chronically worthless or "bad."

Trauma:

The word "trauma" is often used to describe traumatic events, trauma responses, or the longer-term impacts of these events such as PTSD. Here we will break them down separately.

Trauma is the psychological or emotional response to a distressing or disturbing event that overwhelms an individual's ability to cope.

Trauma-Bonding:

Trauma bonding is a powerful hormonal attachment created by abuse and neglect that is alternated with "normal" or loving behavior. This cycle of dependency is at the heart of many relationships in my story, including Randy and my mother, Randy and me, my mother and me.

With each abuse, we are chemically wired to focus solely on getting to the other side. And when the abuser is the person who brings relief, the brain associates them with safety. The brain latches onto the positive experience rather than the impact of staying with the abuser because our body's stress response (fight/flight/freeze/fawn) turns off the part of the brain that can think long-term. This ultimately creates the feeling that you need the abuser to survive and is often mistaken for "love."

The two main ingredients for trauma bonding are a power imbalance and intermittent reinforcement. The greater the power imbalance, the more likely an abused person will develop low self-esteem. When they see themselves as defective, they "need" the person in power to save them.

Intermittent reinforcement is the delivery of an award at inconsistent intervals. An example of this type of conditioning can be seen in gambling. Casinos have long used intermittent reinforcement to help us pour our life savings into their hands, hoping we might finally "win." Intermittent reinforcement is intuitively exploited by people with high levels of narcissism. In conjunction with gaslighting, emotional abuse, and manipulation designed to make us question our reality, the major building blocks for trauma-bonding are formed.

Learning about trauma-bonding allowed me to judge myself a little less for how I had been caught in this cycle. It wasn't because I was broken or didn't deserve love. It was because my nervous system was wired for trauma-bonding in adolescence. My brain made associations based on what I experienced and witnessed: "love" comes with abuse and neglect. We are wired to seek comfort in the face of danger. When safety and comfort cannot be found, we instinctively turn towards abusers to find it.

Trauma Reenactment:

Many traumatized people expose themselves to situations that remind them of their original traumas in an unsuccessful attempt to have a better outcome. This ultimately perpetuates our sense of helplessness and shame.

I repeated the trauma-bonding cycle well into adulthood. Part of the experience I was recreating included the hope that *he will change and then I'll be loved and taken care of.* Just like I hoped as a child. The necessary ingredient to start the cycle *(but this time I'll win)* was attraction to someone who was unavailable, narcissistic, addicted, and so on.

Trauma Responses:

Trauma responses are the body's instinctual reaction to danger. They are unconscious attempts to keep us safe and to maintain connection.

Broadly broken down into four categories: Fight, Flight, Freeze, and Fawn, each response has an adaptive, or healthy expression and a maladaptive, or unhealthy expression.

When we over-rely on one response, it can become fixed. Other healthy responses are difficult to access and we find ourselves perpetually defended, living in a trauma response that we think of as ourselves—our personality.

Fight ranges from assertiveness and expressing healthy boundaries, to explosive anger, bullying and violence.

Flight is to literally flee or stay in perpetual motion. It ranges from efficiency to obsessive/compulsive tendencies, perfectionism, overworking/overdoing, and addiction.

Freeze is numbing or hiding. It's what we think of as classic dissociation. It ranges from being able to rest and find peace, to total avoidance and isolation.

Fawn is a people-pleasing, being of service as a way to avoid vulnerability and feelings. It ranges from being helpful and compassionate to servitude, the abandonment of self for another. Fawning is used after an unsuccessful fight, flight, or freeze attempt.

Most people experience a hybrid of the four main trauma responses. My primary responses are flight (over-working and perfectionism) and fawn (people-pleasing). And one of the ways to find safety outside of these is to lean into the healthy aspects of the fight response—finding a voice, having healthy boundaries, some of the things writing and sharing my story allowed me to practice.

Trauma Therapy:

There are many different modalities for working with trauma, and not every one works for every individual. If you don't find one modality helpful, I encourage you to try another. Some widely researched and utilized trauma therapies are:

Cognitive Behavioral Therapy (CBT), specifically the use of prolonged exposure (PE) and cognitive processing therapy (CPE)

EMDR (Eye Movement Desensitization and Reprocessing)

Internal Family Systems (IFS)

Psychodrama Therapy

Somatic Experiencing (SE)

Traumatic Events:

A traumatic event is an experience in time and space that undermines a person's sense of safety. However, not all traumatic events lead to the development of trauma (the body's inability to fully process the event) or the full criteria for PTSD.

Trigger:

A trigger is a sensory reminder such as a visual cue, noise, smell, or other physical sensation that sets off a memory of a traumatic event.

Triggers can generalize to any characteristic, no matter how small, that resembles or represents a previous trauma. For me, any form of conflict can trigger the feeling of "I'm going to get in trouble," or "I'm about to be grounded."

Sources

American Psychological Association. (n.d.). "Narcissistic Personality Disorder." In *APA dictionary of psychology.* https://dictionary.apa.org/narcissistic-personality-disorder. Accessed June 20, 2022.

Dutton, Don and Painter, Susan L. (1981). "Traumatic Bonding: The Development of Emotional Attachments in Battered Women and Other Relationships of Intermittent Abuse." In *Victimology: An International Journal, vol 6.* https://www.researchgate.net/profile/Donald-Dutton/publication/284119047_Traumatic_bonding_The_development_of_emotional_attachments_in_battered_women_and_other_relationships_of_intermittent_abuse/links/56df531608aee77a15fcfaec/Traumatic-bonding-The-development-of-emotional-attachments-in-battered-women-and-other-relationships-of-intermittent-abuse.pdf?origin=publication_detail. Accessed June 20, 2022.

Van der Kolk, Bessel A. The compulsion to repeat the trauma: re-enactment, revictimization, and masochism. *Psychiatr Clin North Am* 1989;12(2):389-411.

Van der Kolk, Bessel A. *The Body Keeps the Score: Brain, Mind, and Body in the Healing of Trauma.* 2014. Print.

Walker, Pete. "Codependency, Trauma and the Fawn Response." www.pete-walker.com/codependencyFawnResponse.html. Accessed June 20, 2022.

Walker, Pete. "Emotional Flashback Management in the Treatment of Complex PTSD." www.petewalker.com/pdf/emotionalFlashbackManagement.pdf. Accessed June 20, 2022.

Walker, Pete. *Complex PTSD: From Surviving to Thriving.* 2013. Print.

World Health Organization. (2022). "Complex post traumatic stress disorder." In *International classification of diseases for mortality and morbidity statistics (11th Revision).* https://icd.who.int/browse11/l-m/en#/http://id.who.int/icd/entity/585833559. Accessed June 20, 2022.

Resources

For a list of further resources, please visit:

www.IngridClayton.com/Resources

I will continue to add material as I find it useful.

About the Author

Ingrid Clayton, Ph.D., is a clinical psychologist and author of *Recovering Spirituality: Achieving Emotional Sobriety in Your Spiritual Practice.* She is a contributor to *Psychology Today*; her article, "What is Self-Gaslighting?" is considered an Essential Read. Ingrid has been interviewed for countless publications including *Women's Health Magazine* and a guest on numerous podcasts including *The Healing Trauma Podcast.*

While Ingrid has a clinical background, she feels there is no theory, diagnosis, or therapy that can replace the power of shared experience. When she's not making Instagram reels, she enjoys hiking in the mountains and bingeing docuseries with her husband, Yancey.

Ingrid believes, in addition to raising her son, gaining the courage to write this book is her greatest achievement to date.

Visit her on Instagram: @IngridClaytonPhD or on her website: www.IngridClayton.com

Acknowledgements

To my husband, Yancey, who witnessed my process of coming to believe and write my own story, I thank you for telling me to keep going and loving me through it. To everyone who took my calls, many who are not mentioned in the book, I thank you for helping me piece together and validate my experiences. To all of the friends and family who read each version of this book, championing my efforts, I thank you for the unconditional support. To my clients, who have always been my greatest teachers and inspiration, I thank you for showing me such bravery. To the Instagram community of content creators and survivors, you are making the world a better place and I am so grateful. To my editors, Allen Zadoff and Staci Frenes, thank you for distilling my truth in a way that even I could understand it more clearly. To Jillian Shillig, for her creative vision and holding my hand across the finish line, I truly have no words. And to my community of friends, family, sponsors and therapists who have shown me love all along my journey—thank you for loving me to a place where this healing ultimately became possible.

Leave a Review

If you enjoyed this book, I hope you might take a few moments to leave a review on Amazon.

Share it with your friends, family, therapists and teachers so we can raise more awareness about complex trauma and narcissistic abuse.

Thank you!

Made in the USA
Monee, IL
05 November 2022

17024340R00184